Blackburn's
Introduction
to Clinical Radiation
Therapy Physics

Blackburn's Introduction to Clinical Radiation Therapy Physics

Edited by Siamak Shahabi, Ph.D

1989

Medical Physics Publishing Corporation
Madison, Wisconsin

Published by:

Medical Physics Publishing Corporation
27B, 1300 University Ave.
Madison, WI 53706

ISBN: 0-944838-06-5

Library of Congress Cataloging in Publication Data:

Blackburn, Ben.
    Blackburn's introduction to clinical radiation
therapy physics.

    Based on a manuscript by Benjamin Blackburn.
    Bibliography.
    Includes index.
    1. Medical physics. 2. Cancer--Radiotherapy.
I. Shahabi, Siamak. II. Title. III. Title:
Introduction to clinical radiation therapy physics.
R895.B57   1988   615.8'42   88-13905
ISBN 0-944838-06-5

Examples used in this text and data listed in Appendices are for demonstration purposes only. The Editor and Publisher take no responsibility for any damage or harm incurred as a result of use of this information.

Figures on the cover illustrate the isodose distributions for 6 MV photons, 6 x 6 cm field size and 6 MeV electrons, 6 x 6 cone size.

Cover Design by Becky Chapman-Winter

Foreword

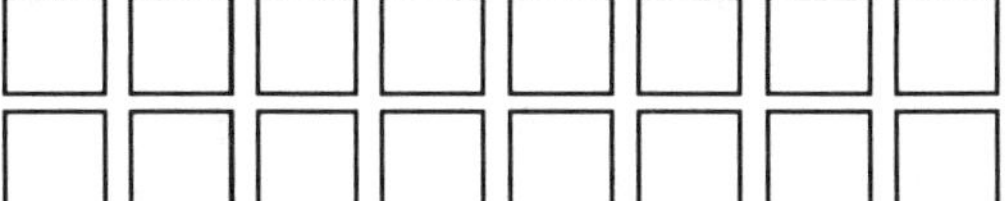

Benjamin E. Blackburn was born in Cincinnati, Ohio on September 12th, 1937 and died of cancer May 28th, 1986. He obtained a B.S. in Physics in 1962 and an M.S. in 1964 in Radiation Physics from the University of Cincinnati. He obtained the latter under Dr. James Kereiakes and in 1965 joined the Department of Radiology (later separating into the Departments of Radiation Oncology and Radiology) of the University of Alabama Hospitals and Clinics, University of Alabama at Birmingham. He was the first resident medical physicist in the state of Alabama. In December 1984 he moved from Birmingham and joined the Department of Radiation Oncology at Jackson-Madison County General Hospital in Jackson, Tennessee.

Ben asked little and gave a lot to his profession, colleagues, friends and family. He commanded the respect of his peers in the Southeast and introduced a number of innovations to the field. He was well known for his willingness to communicate his vast store of radiation therapy physics knowledge. I had the privilege of being his colleague and friend and benefited greatly from my relationship with him. He was widely read and possessed a deep love of nature and the outdoors as well as a keen sense of humor and a subtle wit. Among his hobbies were astronomy, photography, Scrabble, backpacking, and canoeing.

Although Ben was hardworking, a pleasure to be around and work with, and smarter than most of us, he did have one fault. He did not publish many of his innovations or scientific accomplishments. It was sufficient that he did it, and he felt little need to publicize the fact. Also, time might have been a factor as he did virtually all the clinical physics in a busy ($\approx$ 125 patients/day) department by himself.

The majority of the text in this book was written by Ben in the early 1970s for the benefit of his residents. I used his notes to review for my ABR exam in 1975 and suggested then that he publish them. However, it was not until Richard Moreland suggested at the time of Ben's death that arrangements should be made to publish the manuscript that action was taken. A publisher and, more importantly, a competent editor were located and the result is the book before you. It contains much of Ben's personality, and I hope it benefits you as much or more than it benefited Ben's students, residents and colleagues over the past 15 years.

Gary T. Barnes, Ph.D.
Director, Physics Division
Department of Radiology
University of Alabama Hospital and Clinics

Preface

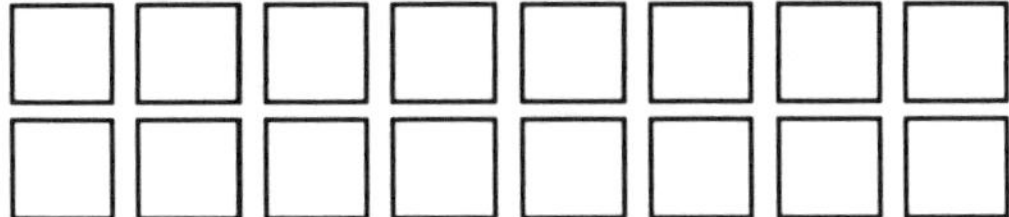

This book is based on a series of lecture notes given by Ben Blackburn on the application of physics to the field of radiation therapy.

This text presents a comprehensive introduction to the basic physics concepts routinely employed in radiation therapy treatment and dose planning. It was designed primarily for teaching residents in radiation therapy; however, it will also be useful as a practical guide for physicists, dosimetrists, and radiation therapy technologists.

When the original notes were written, and while the manuscript was being edited, we tried to keep the reader in mind. We designed the book to be as informative, easy to understand, and useful as possible. The glossary is intended to provide a brief definition of some of the more commonly used terms in the book. It's expansion in future editions will be based on reader input. We would appreciate our readers' opinions and comments so that we can make this book better in future editions.

Siamak Shahabi, Ph.D.
University of Wisconsin-Madison
March 1989

Siamak Shahabi received his Ph.D. in Theoretical Atomic Physics in the Theory of photoionization of open-shell atoms in 1983 from the University of Nebraska-Lincoln. He was a postdoctoral research associate in Atomic Physics at the University of Nebraska-Lincoln during that period. He completed a postdoctoral research fellowship in Therapeutic Radiology in December 1984 at Tufts University School of Medicine, and is now a Clinical Assistant Professor at the University of Wisconsin-Madison Departments of Human Oncology and Medical Physics.

v

Acknowledgements

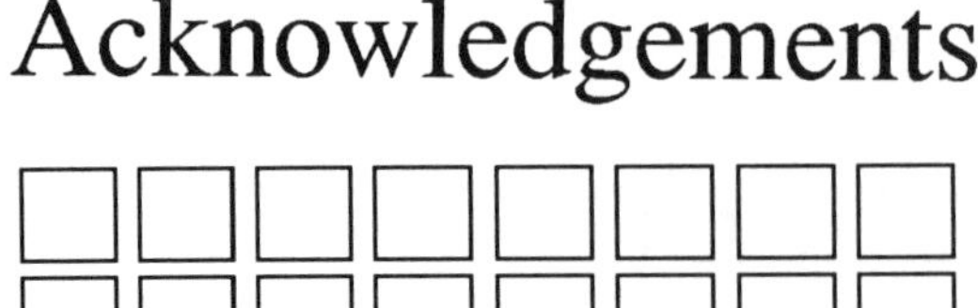

In editing this book I have had the benefit of guidance from a number of people, to whom I am grateful.

My heartfelt thanks go to Dr. John Cameron, Emeritus Professor of Medical Physics, University of Wisconsin-Madison Medical School for reviewing the manuscript and making many insightful comments, and also for providing me with the challenge and opportunity of editing this text.

Thanks also to Jayne Knoche for her careful reading of the text; she pointed out a number of necessary changes. Phyllis Aderholt assisted with typing of the manuscript, and Marla Scogin did a superb job drawing the figures. I would also like to thank Dr. Gary Barnes for his continuing support and time. A warm thanks goes to Mrs. Del Parker, our department secretary. I am deeply indebted to Julie Bogle for her invaluable assitance and technical ability without which this book would have been impossible. Finally, I would like to express my gratitude to the entire Medical Physics Publishing Corporation staff, especially Vicki Stram, Erik Johnson, and Shannon Gilboy, for their invaluable advice, encouragement, and guidance throughout this task.

A special thanks goes to Marcia Heidenreich for her support and patience throughout this project.

S.S.

Contents

Introduction

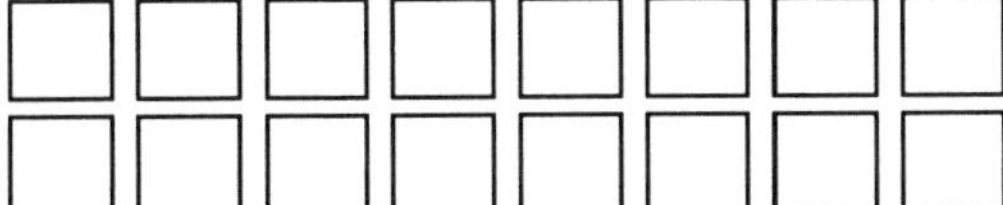

Residents in radiation oncology receive their instruction in physics in basically two categories: theoretical foundations directed toward an understanding of the production and interactions of radiations, and the practical application of those radiations clinically. We will broadly refer to the first category as "theory" and the second as "dosimetry."

Historically the chronological order of presentation in most training programs is an extensive exposure to theory before even a meager introduction to dosimetry. This is a fine idea, and in an ideal world it would undoubtedly be the way to go. Unfortunately, it simply doesn't work.

The resident is called upon to become involved in patient treatment planning very early in his training. If at this point he is armed with the knowledge of how x-rays are produced at the atomic level, and how to calculate the energy content of a single photon if he knows its wavelength, he will find this of minimal help in estimating where to let a linear accelerator beam enter the tissue, or in instructing the technician concerning how long to leave the machine on.

Statements in this book will be given without proof, but with sufficient explanation to enable you to use the concepts in clinical situations and to become conversant with the language. These concepts are of paramount importance - indeed, a thorough understanding of them is necessary to pass the board examinations. The purpose of this book, however, is to make you clinically competent as quickly as possible.

Exposure and Dose

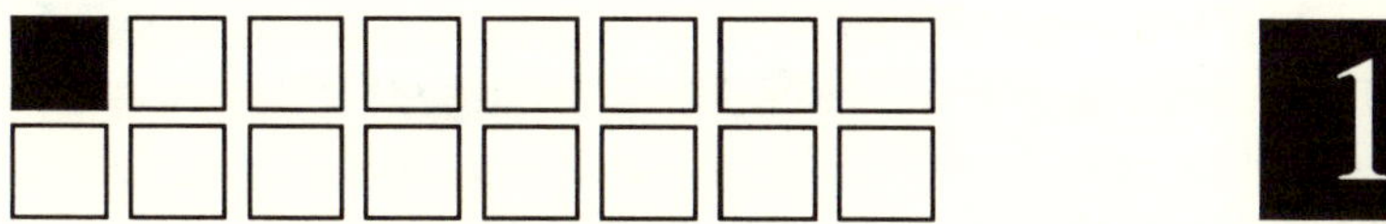

Exposure is a measure of how much x-ray or gamma ray energy is available at a region of interest.[1] It need not be utilized or absorbed, but it must be available for absorption if an absorbing medium is present.

Dose (sometimes called **absorbed dose**) is a measure of how much of this available radiation energy is actually absorbed by a medium which is placed in a radiation beam.[2] The nature of the absorbing medium does not determine the amount of exposure at a point although a medium which absorbs radiation at one point in the beam will reduce exposure at points further along the beam, by removing some of the available radiation.

The nature of the absorber, however, is very important in determining the dose. For example, if a mass of muscle tissue and an equal mass of bone are placed in regions where the available amount of energy (exposure) is the same, the bone may absorb up to four times as much dose as the muscle; or it may absorb a little less, depending on the energy of the radiation. (For the present, think of the energy of the radiation as being equivalent to the penetrating ability.)

An analogy to the concepts of exposure and dose is that of a professor lecturing to a class of students. The information given out by the professor corresponds to exposure, that is, the information available to be learned, whereas the amount absorbed by the listeners corresponds to dose. A bright, alert student will absorb much more than a dull, sleepy student. It is unlikely that either student will absorb all the available knowledge. It is thus with exposure and dose.

The **roentgen (R)** is a unit for quantitatively measuring the amount of exposure.[3] In SI units, exposure is expressed in units of coulombs per kilogram of air. No name is given to 1 C/kg.

The conditions for the measurement of exposure are rigidly specified. Exposure can be measured only in dry air. This does not mean that exposure does not exist in media other than air;

only that you shouldn't attempt to measure exposure in other media. Furthermore, the exposure can only be measured for photons with a fixed energy range. The lower energy limit is set by the fact that the photons must be capable of ionizing air molecules. The upper limit is set at 3 million electron volts or 3 MeV.

To measure exposure, electronic equilibrium must exist in the exposed region.[4,5,6,7] This means that as much electrical charge (due to ionization) must be migrating into the region as out of it. This is necessary if the initially ionized electrons are to be able to expend their energies in a completely natural way by excitations and further ionizations. This can normally be expected only in an extended medium with uniform properties. You will encounter many situations for which this is not so; for example, at the boundary between bone and soft tissue.

The roentgen is 2.58×10^{-4} coulombs of charge liberated per kilogram of air under conditions of electronic equilibrium.* This quantity of charge is either positive or negative. The sum total of all charge will normally be zero, since in an uncharged medium ionization accomplishes only a separation of charge.

What do you do if there is no electronic equilibrium, or if the photon energy exceeds 3 MeV, or if the medium is not air and no air cavity can be inserted, or if the radiation source is charged particles rather than photons? Since the exposure in roentgens cannot be measured in any of these cases, you must accumulate sufficient physical data to calculate the absorbed dose.[8] The SI unit of dose is the gray (Gy), which is 1 joule (J) of energy absorbed per kilogram of absorbing medium. The other common unit of dose is the rad ("radiation absorbed dose"); 1 rad = 0.01 Gy = 1 cGy (centigray).[9] You will often calculate a dose in cGy from the exposure measured in roentgens.

Since the roentgen suffers from the many limitations listed above and the rad does not, why bother with the roentgen at all? The roentgen has only one advantage over the rad, in that it can often be measured easily. Nevertheless, you can get by completely without reference to the roentgen, and some day it may join the dodo bird and the brontosaurus.

The concept of exposure will eventually be replaced by the "kerma" (kinetic energy released in the medium). Kerma measures energy transferred to charged particles, per unit mass of the medium, and uses the same unit as dose. Air kerma corresponds to exposure. Since kerma has not yet come into general use, we will not discuss subtleties in its definition.

Dose corresponds to points, not volumes. It is important to recognize that the concept of dose holds true only for individual

---

* The roentgen is also equal to one electrostatic unit (esu) of charge per cm^3 of air at 0° centigrade and one atmosphere of pressure.

points in the irradiated medium. You may state that you are going to give an entire tumor a 60 Gy dose in six weeks, but it would be practically impossible to do so. Even with extreme care and planning, the dose at two points within a few centimeters of each other will differ by several percent. You may say, however, that the dose on a central ray at a depth of seven centimeters will be 60 Gy. The target specified here is a point, and not a volume.

But how can you reconcile the concept of dose at a point with the definition of dose, which is energy absorbed in a given mass of tissue (corresponding to a specific volume)? Consider the hypothetical case of a gram of tissue receiving a total of 10^{-3} J (0.001 joule) of energy. One gram (10^{-3} kg) of tissue equals one cm^3, a definite volume. The absorbed dose is 10^{-3} J/10^{-3} kg, which equals 1 J/kg, which is the definition of 1 Gy. (You don't need to use the energy absorbed by a whole kilogram, when in fact the dose will usually not be constant over such a large region.)

Figure 1.1

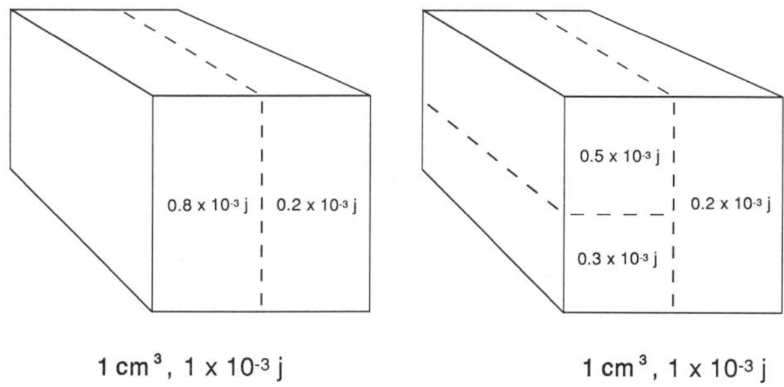

But now suppose that you divide that cm^3 of tissue in half and find that the left half absorbed 0.8 x 10^{-3} J, and the right half only 0.2 x 10^{-3} J (the initial total of 1 x 10^{-3} J over the entire gram). You would calculate the dose of the left side as:

$$\frac{0.8 \times 10^{-3}\,J}{0.5 \times 10^{-3}\,kg} = 1.6\;Gy$$

Now suppose further that the upper half of this half (1/4 gram) absorbed 0.5 x 10^{-3} J, and the lower half absorbed 0.3 x 10^{-3} J (still 0.8 x 10^{-3} J in the half gram).

The dose to the upper half of the half would be:

$$\frac{0.5 \times 10^{-3}\,J}{0.25 \times 10^{-3}\,kg} = 2\;J/kg = 2\;Gy$$

If you are primarily interested in the upper left quadrant of the gram, the initial estimate of 1 Gy based on 10^{-3} J per gram already involves an error of 100%.

You could continue this division of the original gram into smaller and smaller volumes and recalculate the dose as the energy locally absorbed divided by the mass of the tiny volume, giving us an answer in joule per kilogram, or Gy. You could continually divide this tiny volume until it encompassed a single cell, which for practical purposes would constitute a point in the tissue. At this point you might find the dose within the cell to be 20 or 30 Gy, instead of the 1 Gy we initially assumed. The cell would respond as if it had absorbed 30 Gy instead of 1, thus demonstrating that dose truly corresponds to individual points rather than volumes.

Consider now the dose to two irradiated patients. In one patient, a 1 x 1 cm field centered on the body such that the point at midline receives 10 Gy. The entire body of the other patient is irradiated with a uniform radiation field so that the same midline point receives 10 Gy. There is an obvious difference in the two situations; namely there will be very little permanent damage to the first patient, whereas the second patient will almost certainly die within a few weeks from radiation effects.

The difference here is not a difference of dose. The prescribed dose in both cases is 10 Gy. You obviously need some factor in addition to dose in order to evaluate total response of the tissue. This factor is the **integral dose**, which is a measure of the total energy absorbed by the irradiated medium.[10,11] Integral dose is the product of the dose to tiny volumes times the masses of those tiny volumes, added up over the entire irradiated medium.

The SI unit of integral dose is the kg Gy (1 kg Gy = 1 J). The older unit is the gram rad (1 gram rad = 10^{-5} J).

The calculation of integral dose is an extremely time consuming and difficult (if not impossible) task, as might be imagined from our earlier discussion involving the variation of dose from point to point within one gram of tissue. A number of methods of approximating the integral dose are available, and we will look at these later.

It should be pointed out, however, that you are rarely interested in the exact integral dose in any specific case. Often you will compare modes of treatment and types of therapy in order to minimize integral dose. For example, a specific clinical problem can be treated with a single field, an opposing pair, multiple fields, or arc therapy. Concerns over minimizing integral dose also influence the choice of therapy. For example, a deep-seated tumor can be given 60 Gy using orthovoltage beams, cobalt-60 gamma rays, or megavoltage x-rays from a linear accelerator. The integral dose would be highest from the orthovoltage technique and lowest from the highest energy linear accelerator beam, if all other factors are equal.

As previously stated, even if you know the exposure in roentgens to which a medium is exposed, you will calculate the dose in order to evaluate biological or other effects. There are many ways to do this. The simplest method is to multiply the number of roentgens by a quantity referred to as the **f-factor**.[12] The dose in cGy = (exposure in roentgens) · (f), where f is typically in rad/R, for a specified photon energy in a specified medium. The value of the f-factor depends on the energy of the photons and on the nature of the absorber. There are published tables of f-factors in various biological media as a function of photon energy. Figure 1.2 shows the variation in f-factors for compact bone and striated muscle tissue from 0.01 MeV to 3.0 MeV. Notice that the graph cannot extend above the set limit of 3 MeV.

Some f-factors for various materials can be found in Johns and Cunningham, 4th Edition, table A-4, page 739.

Figure 1.2

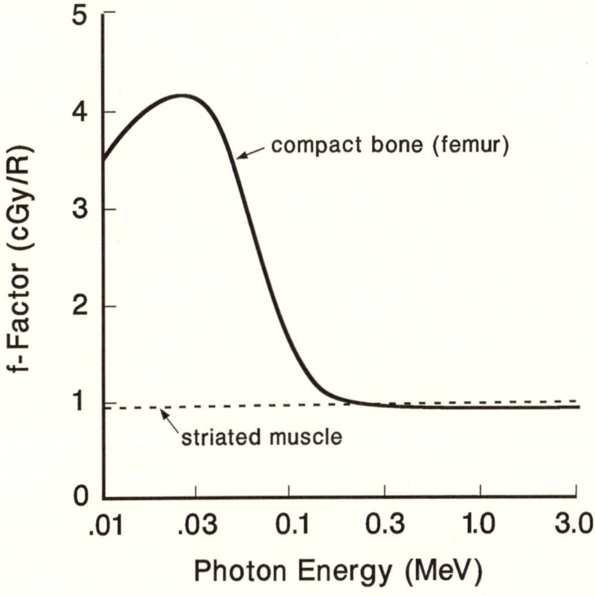

References

1. *Radiation Quantities and Units,* Report 19, International Commission on Radiation Units and Measurement, Bethesda, 1971, p. 8.
2. Ibid., p. 7.
3. Ibid.
4. Attix, F.H. *Introduction to Radiological Physics and Radiation Dosimetry,* John Wiley & Sons, New York, 1986, Chapter 4.
5. Meredith, W.J. & Massey, J.B. *Fundamental Physics of Radiology,* 3rd Edition, John Wright & Sons, Bristol, 1976, pp. 449-451.
6. *Determination of Absorbed Dose in a Patient Irradiated by Beams of X or Gamma Rays in Radiotherapy,* Report 24, International Commission on Radiation Units, Bethesda, 1976, p. 52.
7. Johns, H.E. & Cunningham, J.R. *The Physics of Radiology*, 4th Edition, Charles C. Thomas, Springfield, 1983, pp. 220-223.
8. See glossary for definition.
9. See glossary for more detailed definition.
10. Johns & Cunningham, pp. 402-405.
11. Mayneord, W.V. "The Measurement of Radiation for Medical Purposes," *Proc Phys Soc* 54:405, 1942.
12. Johns & Cunningham, p. 739.

Inverse Square Law

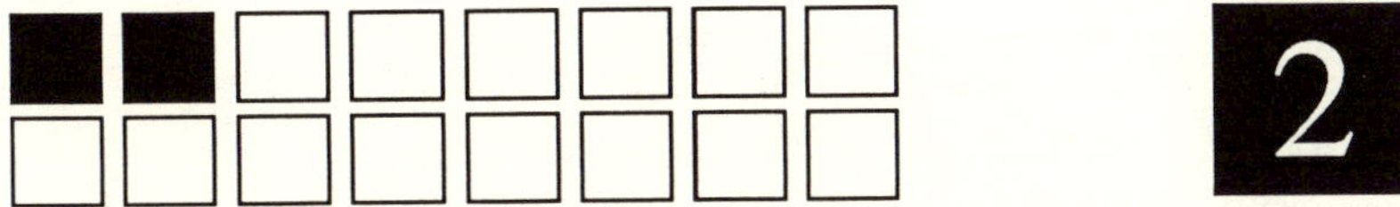

2

The further you get from a radiation source, the less intense is the beam. If this were not true, each of the distant stars would give us as much light as the sun and we would be quickly cooked.

If you double your distance from the source, the exposure becomes one fourth as much; if you triple the distance, the exposure is one ninth as much, and so on. This results in an inverse square proportion between intensity and distance:

$$\left(\frac{I_1}{I_2} = \left(\frac{d_2}{d_1}\right)^2 \right)$$

where I_1 is the intensity at a point whose distance from the source is d_1, and I_2 is the intensity at a point whose distance from the source is d_2.[1,2] Note that the subscripts are inverted on opposite sides of the equation, and the right side is squared whereas the left side is not. Hence the term **inverse square law**.

Example 2.1:

> The intensity at a distance of 40 cm from a point source is 90 R/minute. What is the intensity at a distance of 100 cm from this source?

Let I_2 = 90 R/min, and thus d_2 = 40 cm. I_1 is asked for, and d_1 = 100 cm.

$$\frac{I_1}{I_2} = \frac{I_1}{90\,R/min} = \left(\frac{d_2}{d_1}\right)^2 = \left(\frac{40cm}{100cm}\right)^2 = (0.4)^2 = 0.16$$

$$I_1 = 0.16 \times 90\,R/min = 14.4\,R/min$$

Note the term "point source" in the above example. The inverse square law is strictly true only when the radiation source is a geometric point. Since no such source exists in nature, what good is the inverse square law? The answer is that the law provides a very good approximation if the source "appears" as a "point" when viewed from where the intensity or exposure is measured. Considering the distant stars as point sources leads to no measurable error. Even though many of those stars are hundreds of millions of miles in diameter, our most powerful telescopes see them only as geometrical points.

How far away must the source be before it seems like a point? A more appropriate question is how far away must the source be for the inverse square law to involve an acceptably small error? A rule of thumb to remember is if the maximum dimension of the source is L, then at distances of 4L or greater, the inverse square law will result in errors of less than 2%. If you are, for example, 10L away from the source, the error is much less than 1%. Teletherapy sources range in diameter from 0.2 cm to about 3.0 cm, and the points of interest are normally further away than 50 cm. Can you infer from this that teletherapy sources will follow the inverse square law with 99% accuracy?   Not necessarily, since other factors are involved in calculating accuracy, such as scattering from the collimator, air scattering and absorption, etc. However, most high energy teletherapy sources (cobalt-60, linear accelerators, etc.) obey the inverse square law to within about 2% over with the range that is normally used.

References

1. Sprawls, P. *The Physical Principles of Diagnostic Radiology,* University Park Press, Baltimore, 1977.
2. Halliday, D. & Resnick, R. *Fundamentals of Physics*, 2nd Edition, John Wiley & Sons, New York, 1981, p. 301.

External Beam Radiation Sources

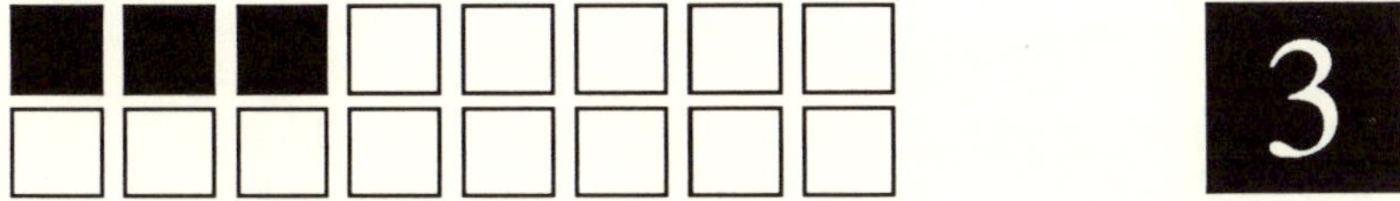

3

There are several ways to express the relative penetrating abilities (sometimes called "hardness") of ionizing radiations. You may simply state the peak excitation voltage for x-rays, which means the potential difference that electrons are made to "fall" through in order to produce x-rays.[1] This voltage is normally expressed in kilovolts (kVp) or megavolts (MV). In general, the higher the kVp or MV, the greater the penetrating ability.[2,3,4] This trend tends to reverse itself for extremely high energy x-rays, but in body tissues this reversal occurs above the clinically useful voltage range.

You can also specify relative penetrating ability by the half value layer (HVL) of the beam.[5] The HVL is the thickness of a specified material which reduces the intensity of a beam to 1/2 its initial value. The material used must be specified. The statement "The HVL of this beam is 3 mm" is ambiguous, whereas "HVL = 3 mm of copper" is not. In certain voltage ranges, the material may be understood without specifically stating it. For example, if you stated that you are using a superficial beam with HVL = 1 mm, then those familiar with superficial therapy would assume that the HVL was measured in aluminum. It is not good practice to depend upon such assumptions.

Table 3.1 lists some teletherapy sources with their excitation voltages, typical half value layers, and materials in which the HVL is traditionally measured.[6]

Grenz Ray Therapy involves very soft radiations, such that the first few layers of cells encountered have a significant effect on beam intensity. Such therapy is not often used these days, except by a few dermatologists.

Contact Therapy also involves soft x-rays and is again not used often, except by dermatologists.

Superficial Therapy x-rays are useful in treating skin cancers which involve depths of 5 or 6 mm of tissue. An alternative to this mode is electron beam therapy.

Table 3.1

Teletherapy Type	Excitation Voltages	HVL
Grenz rays	0 - 25 kVp	a few sheets of cellophane
Contact therapy	25 - 50 kVp	0.1 - 0.5 mm Al
Superficial therapy	50 - 150 kVp	0.5 - 6 mm Al
Intermediate voltage	150 - 200 kVp	0.25 - 2 mm Cu
Orthovoltage	200 - 400 kVp	2 - 5 mm Cu
Teleisotope	*	several mm of lead
Megavoltage	> 1 MV	several mm of lead

Intermediate Voltage Therapy is useful for lesions up to a few cm deep.

Orthovoltage Therapy can be used for deeper lesions, and originally was called "deep therapy." It involves a greater risk of morbidity to overlying healthy tissues than does modern teleisotope or megavoltage equipment. Often intermediate voltage and orthovoltage are lumped together as a single category under the name orthovoltage.

Teleisotope Therapy is specifically suited to deep lesions. The isotopes cobalt-60 and cesium-137 are primarily used. Cesium-137, however, is uncommon.

Megavoltage Therapy, again specifically suited to deep lesions, involves very hard x-rays. Older devices generating these radiations were the resonant transformer, the Van de Graaff generator, and the betatron. While a few of these devices are still in use, modern megavoltage therapy generally employs the linear accelerator.

In addition to the above sources of photon radiations, certain particle radiations are used in teletherapy (external beam therapy):

Electron beams are foremost among these.

Neutrons seem to have a definite advantage over other radiations for treating hypoxic tissues.[7,8,9,10,11] Their use is experimental and they will not be discussed in this book.

Pi mesons or pions were used experimentally for a few years.[12] Installations for their production are extremely expensive, and a considerable technical professional staff is required. Their use is not likely to become widespread in the foreseeable future.

Proton beams have certain definite advantages.[13,14,15,16] While still quite expensive and requiring considerable technical expertise, they may find considerable use in the future in a few major institutions.

---

* No excitation voltages are expressed for teleisotope radiations since these are gamma rays coming from radioactive materials. An example is cobalt-60 which emits gamma rays of 1.17 and 1.33 Mev, whose photons have an average energy of 1.25 MeV. A cobalt-60 beam has about the same penetrating ability as a 3 MV x-ray beam.

References

1. Johns, H.E. & Cunningham, J.R. *The Physics of Radiology*, 4th Edition, Charles C. Thomas, Springfield, 1983, Chapter 2.
2. Hendee, W.R. *Radiation Therapy Physics,* 2nd Edition, Year Book Medical Publishers, Chicago, 1979, pp. 94-96.
3. Khan, F.M. *The Physics of Radiation Therapy*, Williams & Wilkins, Baltimore, 1984, p. 210.
4. Johns & Cunningham, pp. 362-364.
5. Ibid., pp. 33, 137, 270.
6. *Structural Shielding Design and Evaluation for Medical Use of X-Rays and Gamma Rays of Energies Up To 10 MeV*, NCRP Report 49, National Council on Radiation Protection and Measurements, Washington, D.C., 1976, pp. 33-34.
7. Catterall, M. "The Treatment of Advanced Cancer by Fast Neutrons from the Medical Research Council's Cyclotron at Hammersmith Hospital, London," *Eur J Can* 10: 343-347, 1974.
8. Laramore, G.E. et al. "Fast Neutron Radiotherapy for Locally Advanced Prostate Cancer: Results of an RTOG Randomized Study," *Int J Radiat Oncol, Biol Phys* 11: 1621-1627, 1985.
9. Pelton, J.G. et al. "Fast Neutron Radiotherapy for Soft Tissue Sarcomas," *Am J Clin Oncol* 9:397-400, 1986.
10. Stone, R.S. "Neutron Therapy and Specific Ionization," *Am J Roentgen* 59:771-785, 1948.
11. Griffin, B.R. & Stewart, G.R. *Fast Neutron Radiotherapy: An Overview of Medical Dosimetry*, Vol. 13, 1988, pp. 19-21.
12. Goodman, G.B. et al. "Preparatory Clinical Studies of Pi-Mesons at TRIUMF," *Radiation Research* 104:s279-s284, 1985.
13. Austin-Seymour, M. et al. "Progress in Low-Let Heavy Particle Therapy: Intracranial and Paracranial Tumors and Uveal Melanomas," *Radiation Research* 104:s219-s226, 1985.
14. Hiroshi, T. et al. "Proton Therapy in Japan," *Radiation Research* 104:s235-s243, 1985.
15. Suit, H.O. et al. "Clinical Experience and Expectation with Proton and Heavy Ions," *Int J Radiat Oncol Biol Phys* 3:115-125, 1977.
16. Duttenhaver, J.D. et al. "Protons or Megavoltage X-Rays as Boost Therapy for Patients Irradiated for Localized Prostatic Carcinoma," *Cancer* 51:1599-1604, 1983.

Characteristics of External Beam Photon Fields

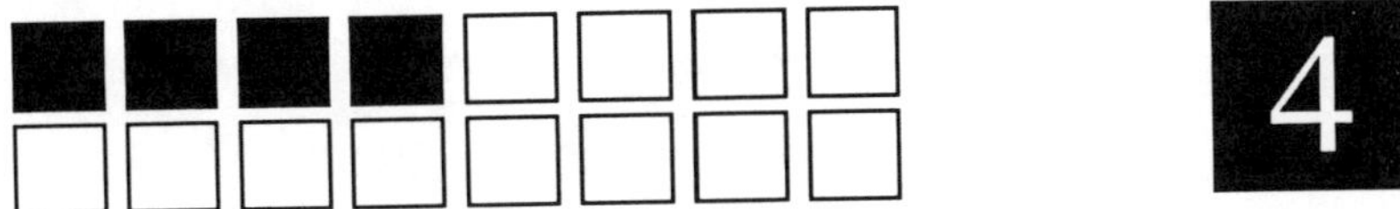

4

A. Dose Buildup
B. Dose vs. Depth as a Function of Energy
C. Exit Dose Reduction
D. Dose at Points Off the Central Ray
E. Definition of Field Size

A.

Dose Buildup

Energy is carried into the irradiated tissue primarily by the radiation coming from the source. However, the energy is distributed in the tissue primarily by secondary electrons set in motion by this primary radiation. The dose distribution depends mostly on the range of these secondary electrons.

For soft radiation, such as Grenz rays and superficial x-rays, these secondaries are immediately set in motion at the surface, and travel immediately in all directions, but their energies are quickly absorbed. Below the surface, there is less and less primary radiation due to the lack of penetrating ability of the original radiation. Thus for a soft radiation, the maximum absorbed dose for a single field occurs at the skin.

For higher energy radiation, the number of secondaries tends to build up more slowly primarily due to longer range of the electrons. In addition, the secondary particles have less tendency to "bounce away" sideways; they tend to be set in motion more or less in the same direction the primary was traveling.

Pretend that the tissue in Figure 4.1 has imaginary layers and is being irradiated by a high energy photon beam. Suppose that we consider only the forward recoil secondaries, and that on the average these are capable of traveling to depths of up to four layers before losing all of their energy. Dose to an individual layer will depend on: (a) electrons set in motion within that layer

Figure 4.1

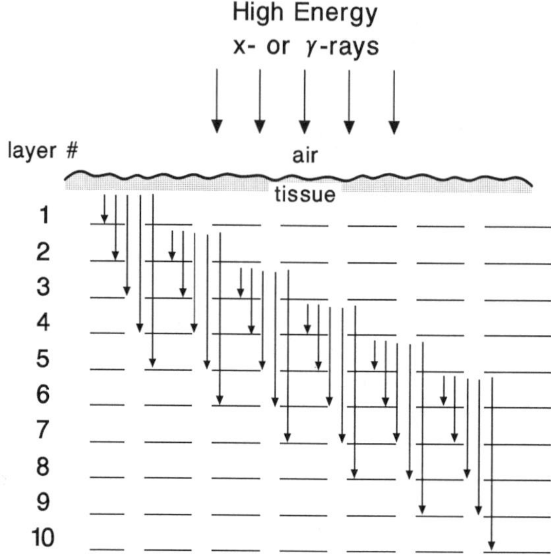

and depositing their energy in the same layer, and (b) electrons which were set in motion above, but deposit their energy in this layer. To simplify this example, let us assume that the primary is equally intense in the first several layers. For a hard radiation, and thin imaginary layers, this is close to the truth.

Let's assume that:

(1) there are no electrons coming from air, only photons (approximation);

(2) we can ignore the loss of energy of photons in the top 6 layers (approximation);

(3) the range of secondary electrons is up to 4 layers.

Consider layer one (1). Dose here is due to only category (a) electrons, since none are entering from above. In layer two (2), we have electrons in category (a), and also some electrons from layer (1). In layer three (3), we have electrons in category (a), and electrons from both layers (1) and (2). Obviously, the dose in layer (3) is greater than in layer (2), which in turn was greater than in layer (1). In layer (4) we have category (a) electrons and electrons from layers (1), (2), (3) and (4), and the dose is greater still. In layer (5), we now have category (a) electrons and electrons from layers (1), (2), (3), and (4) and the dose is greater again. In layer (6) we have category (a) electrons and electrons from layers (2), (3), (4), and (5), but not from layer (1), since they have sufficient energy to penetrate through only four layers. Thus, given the simplifying assumption, the dose will not be greater in layer (6) than in layer (5), since both have category (a) electrons and electrons from only four overlying layers. In actual fact, there will be slightly less dose in layer (6), due to the fact that it is receiving slightly less primary because of attenuation in the overlying layers. In layer (5), we reach electronic equilibrium. This is referred to as the **depth of maximum dose** (d_{max}) or as the **buildup depth**, and depends on field size and the energy of the primary radiation.[1,2,3,4] The buildup depth is the depth at the point on central axis of the field at which **maximum dose** (D_{max}) occurs. The buildup depth is only a fraction of a millimeter for orthovoltage radiation, about 5 mm for cobalt-60 gamma rays, about 1 cm for 4 MV x-rays, and about 2.5 cm for 10 MV x-rays. The region from the surface (skin) to the maximum dose is also known as the **buildup region**.

Also, the relative or percent dose at the skin surface is less for radiations having a greater buildup depth, i.e., higher energy radiations. For example, for the same field size, the skin dose for a superficial field will be 100% (buildup point is on the skin), where the buildup point is defined as the point on the central axis at which the dose is maximum. For an orthovoltage field, skin dose may be 97% of D_{max} at a point just beneath the skin. While the skin dose is only 40% of D_{max} for a cobalt-60 field, where D_{max} occurs at 5 mm. Skin dose may be as low as 25% for a 4 MV beam, and perhaps 18% for a 10 MV beam. The lower skin dose for high energy radiation is called **skin sparing**.

The percent skin dose also varies with field size; it is greater for larger field sizes due to additional scattered radiation from

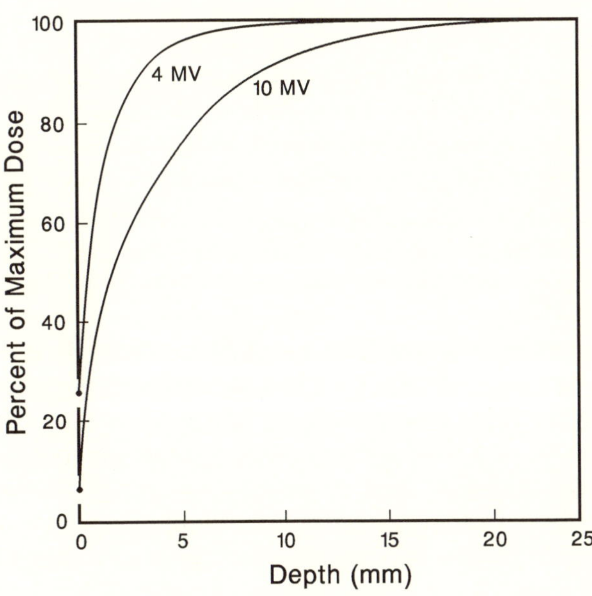

Figure 4.2. Dose buildup characteristics of x-ray beams from Clinac-4 (CL-4) and Clinac-18 (CL-18). Measured with single-crystal layers of lithium fluoride for 15 x 15 cm field sizes at 79 cm SSD (CL-4) and 100 cm SSD (CL-18).

the collimation and more backscattered radiation from the patient. The percent skin dose will also be increased by a blocking tray or other object close to the skin.

The skin dose is a very difficult thing to measure, since even for a high energy radiation, it may double within the first millimeter; thus the measuring device must be extremely thin, and not many methods of measurement are suitable.

Contrary to the earlier example, buildup is not linear. For example, if the skin dose is 24%, and the maximum buildup occurs at one cm, you might suppose that at 5 mm the dose would be 62% (halfway between 24% and 100%. Figure 4.2 shows this to be a serious error, since for the Clinac-4, the dose is 96%.

It is important to be aware not only of the percent skin dose and the depth at which buildup occurs, but also of the rapidity with which the dose approaches maximum buildup, particularly when critical tissues lie near the depth of maximum dose.

Note, for example, that although the nominal d_{max} for the Clinac-4 is at one cm, the dose is 90% of maximum at only 3 mm depth, and for the 10 MV beam from the Clinac-18, whose d_{max} is at about 2.5 cm, 90% dose occurs at 7.5 mm.

Reduction or loss of skin sparing can occur either intentionally or unintentionally.[5,6] An example calling for intentional reduction of skin sparing would be where part of the target volume is at or very near the skin, yet other aspects of the problem indicate the advisability of high energy photons. In order to prevent serious underdosing of the surface, bolus may be placed on the skin at the involved site.[7] If this bolus has about the same density and average atomic number as the skin, the radiation will not distinguish between it and the patient. For example, if one cm of bolus is placed on the skin in a 4 MV field, buildup will occur in the bolus and the maximum dose will be on the skin surface.

Please note that it is not necessary to use a bolus thickness equal to the buildup depth. A dose at the skin surface of 90 to 95% of maximum is usually adequate. For example, instead of adding a bolus of 25 mm thickness on the surface for a 10 MV beam to achieve 100% dose at the surface, you could add 10 mm and achieve 95%.

It is important to recognize that this bolus must be taken into account in the treatment plan as if it were tissue. For example, if you want to deliver a prescribed dose of 60 Gy to a tissue depth of 8 cm, and you have added 1 cm of bolus, you should proceed as if the tissue depth is actually 9 cm. The effective source to surface distance (SSD) is the distance to the top of the bolus.

Undesirable loss of skin sparing occurs whenever material

covers the skin in the treatment area. For example, if a patient cannot remain motionless during treatment, an immobilizing cast of plastic or some other material must be used. This cast may cover a portion or all of the treatment field. A skin reaction beneath the cast should be expected. Another example is that of a prosthesis or cast which cannot be removed without great risk.

The most drastic example occurs when metal is near or in actual contact with the skin inside the field. This may be due to field shaping blocks placed too near the skin (or a device such as a trachea tube which has not been removed). In cases like this, the skin reaction can be even greater than it would be if the normal buildup occurred on the skin, or in other words, the percent skin dose exceeds the dose at d_{max}. The extra reaction is due to an intense rain of electrons coming from the metal as a result of the increased photoelectric effect.

Skin sparing is also reduced whenever the radiation enters the skin nonperpendicularly. The maximum dose occurs at the usual depth, but that depth is measured along the rays, and is equal to the depth beneath the skin only in the case of a perpendicular beam (Figure 4.3).

Figure 4.3

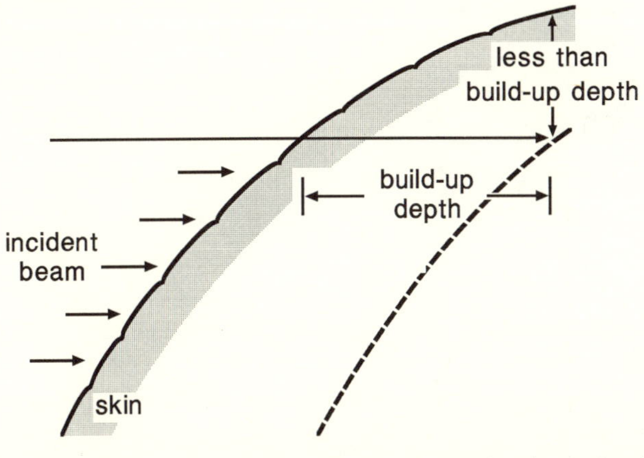

Obviously this effect is most pronounced when the beam is tangent to the skin, in which case the maximum dose occurs virtually on the surface, although no bolus is present (Figure 4.4).

Figure 4.4

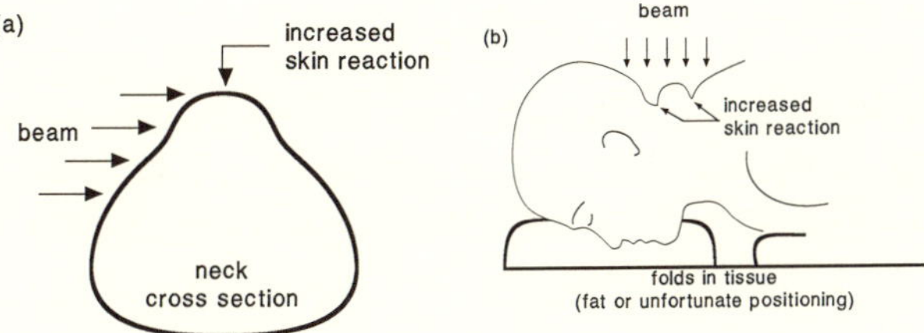

Loss of electronic equilibrium, or regaining of skin sparing, can also pose a clinical problem. Since "buildup" as we have discussed it is a buildup of electrons, and electrons are attenuated much more rapidly than photons, electronic equilibrium will be lost by the introduction of air cavities. In this case, electrons are being removed by the air, but are not being efficiently replaced by more photon reactions (Figure 4.5).

For a quantitative view of this phenomenon, see Figure 4.6.

Figure 4.5

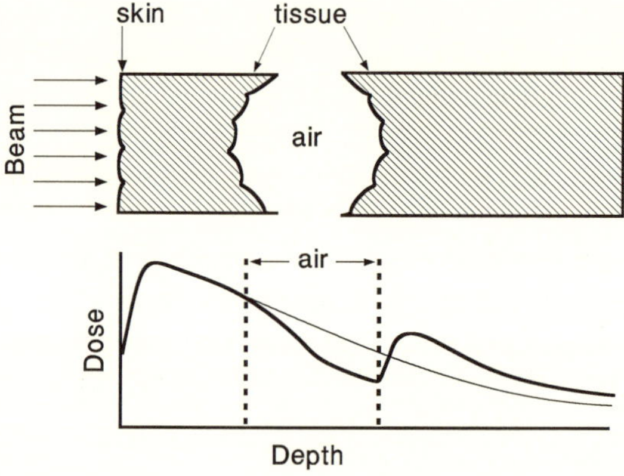

Figure 4.6

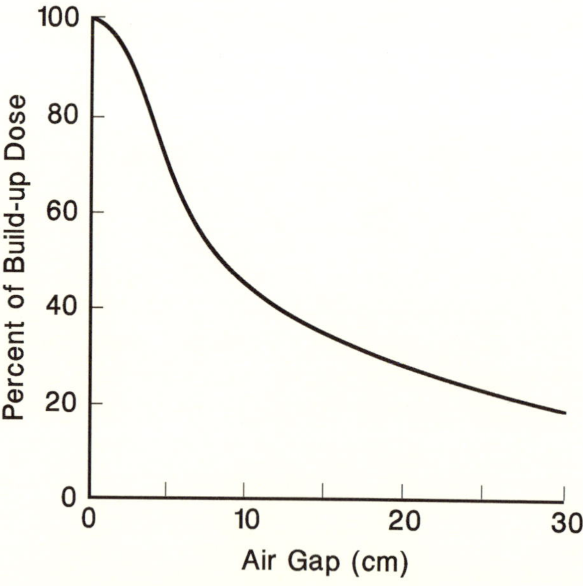

To some extent, air cavities help determine the placement of field shaping blocks. The blocks and/or the plastic tray supporting the blocks should be far enough from the skin to regain a reasonable amount of skin sparing, since electronic equilibrium will occur in the block support. A 15 cm gap is recommended.[8,9] This is not feasible for some cobalt-60 units because of an extended collimator. A gap of 10 cm is sufficient to avoid serious skin reaction in nearly all cases with such a unit. However, for gaps of less than 8 cm, heightened skin reactions appear frequently.

B.

Depth Dose Data as a Function of Energy

Figure 4.7 contains much information for the evaluation of the merits and shortcomings of various treatment modes. The graphs represent photon beams entering a water medium under the following conditions:

(a) perpendicular entry;

(b) "semi-infinite" depth; i.e., enough water depth exists beyond the measured points so that if more depth were added, it would not affect the measurements (usually about 15 cm beyond the last measured point);

(c) depth vs. dose on central ray;

(d) no inhomogeneities in the irradiated medium;

(e) 10 x 10 cm field at the depth of maximum dose.

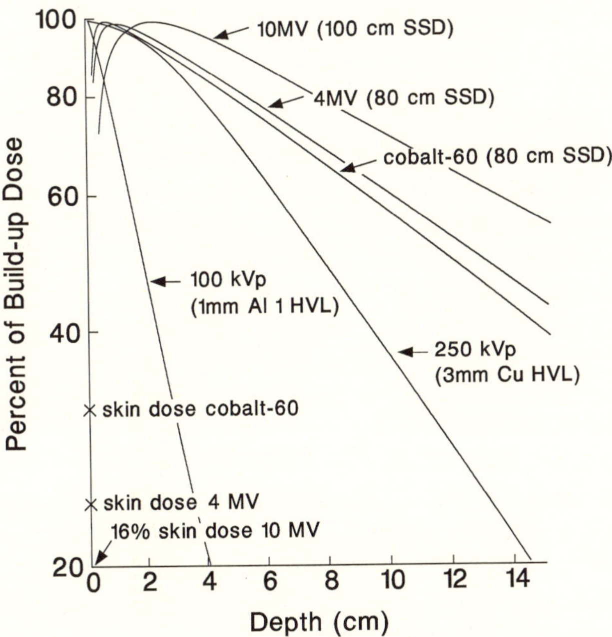

Figure 4.7. Dose versus depth for a range of clinically useful photon energies.

Water is used because it is nearly "tissue-equivalent" in terms of effective atomic number, mass density, and electron density.

Note that the horizontal scale (depth) is linear (equal divisions) whereas the vertical scale is logarithmic. It is useful to present depth vs. dose curves on a semi-logarithmic graph due to the exponential law of absorption. However, this law applies only to monochromatic (single energy) radiations. Due to the fact that most of these beams have a spectrum of photon energies, and, in addition, the ratio of primary to scattered radiation changes, these depth dose curves will never be straight lines on such a graph.

C.

Depth Dose Data as a Function of Energy

As pointed out previously, the graphs of Figure 4.7 assume a semi-infinite medium, which implies a considerable amount of tissue-like medium after the last point of interest. This is obviously not the case in a great many clinical situations. The patient is positioned on a rather thin table, and if the deepest point of interest is the exit surface of the skin, there is not more than one or two centimeters (cm) of material after this point. Since the tables and graphs you will use almost invariably assume a semi-infinite medium, how can dose be estimated in the above situations when a semi-infinite medium is not present?

The dose contributed to each point is due to both primary and scattered radiation. The scattered component partly consists of backward-scattered radiation. In the absence of a scattering medium (other than air) beyond the point of interest, this backscattered radiation will not be present to contribute to the dose. Thus the dose will be less than that estimated from standard tables. It would be extremely difficult to present tabular data indicating how much less, since this depends on: (a) radiation type, (b) source to surface (skin) distance (SSD), (c) field size, (d) patient thickness, and (e) nature of patient support.

In general, however, the average patient supported on an average couch, irradiated by a 15 x 15 cm field from a cobalt-60 unit at an SSD of 80 cm, will experience about a 6% underdose at the exit surface if the standard tables are used. This refers to 6% of the dose estimated at the exit point and not 6% of the maximum dose. For example, if a 1 Gy dose is given at d_{max} and 30 cGy is estimated from a table as the exit dose, the actual exit dose will be about 28.2 cGy (not 24 cGy).

For a radiation harder than cobalt-60 (for energies greater than 4 MV), this error will not be as great, since less radiation is backscattered with harder radiations. On the other hand, the error will be greater for softer radiations (orthovoltage, superficial), but exit dose is rarely a concern in such cases.

Figure 4.8

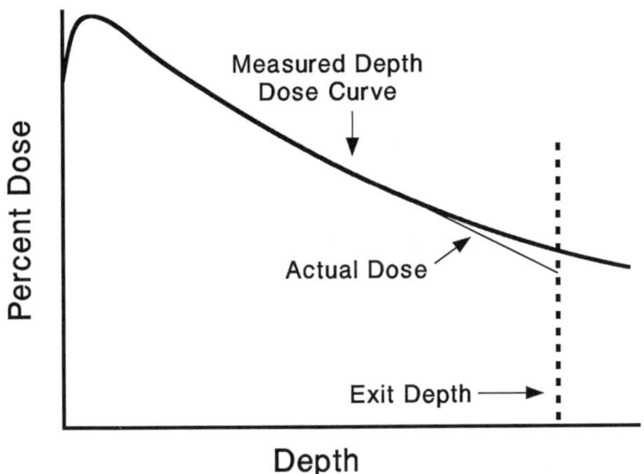

D.
Dose at Points off the Central Ray

Thus far our interest has concerned points along a single line directly down the center of the field. This one dimensional picture is often inadequate, since an actual clinical situation exists in three dimensions, even when only a single field is being used.

The relationship between the doses on and off the central ray is extremely complex, depending on type of radiation, SSD, angle of central ray to skin surface, nature of collimator, field size, penumbra, source size, presence of beam flattening filters, and field shaping blocks.[10]

Because of the complex relationship, no mathematical technique can truly predict the actual dose distribution. A few approximate techniques are available for computer treatment planning. Even so, these techniques must be augmented by a considerable amount of measurement.

The only sure way of determining dose off the central axis is by measurement. These measurements need to be repeated for the many combinations of parameters listed above. Obviously, this could take a great deal of time. If you restrict your measurements to perpendicular beams with no blocking for a particular machine with known collimation, source size, and flattening filter, you can gather the necessary measurements in a reasonable amount of time. From these data, estimates of dose can be made when the beam is not perpendicular to the skin and when blocks are used. It is possible to keep the error in such estimates manageably small if great care is taken. However, you must understand that these are approximations, and there will always be some error, so you must eliminate error at each step where it is possible to do so.

There are several methods of presenting dose data for points off the central ray. Dose profiles are graphs of dose versus distance from the central ray, at fixed depths [Figures 4.9 (a), (b)]. Dose profiles may be used for clinical dosimetry, but their use is somewhat limited by the fact that they correspond to single fixed depths and are only two dimensional.

Figure 4.9 (a). Dose profiles for cobalt-60 10 x 10 cm field, at d_{max} and at 10 cm depth. Figure 4.9 (b). Dose profile for 4 MV x-rays 10 x 10 cm field. Note the "horns."

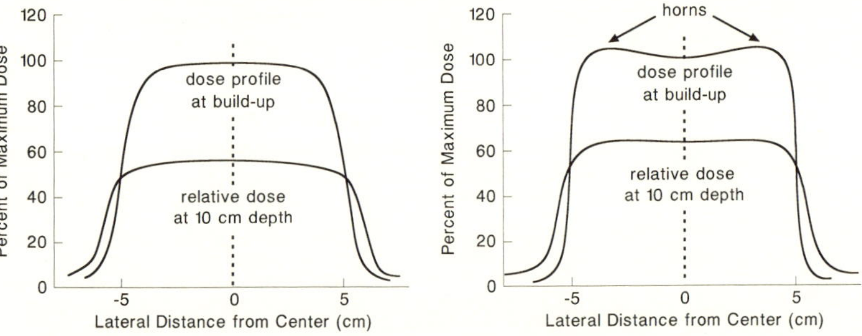

Some aspects of the dose profiles of Figure 4.9 are worthy of special note. Three distinct regions become apparent as you move outward from the central ray in either direction.

First, there is a broad region in which the dose changes slowly from point to point, increasing or decreasing only slightly. This is called the **full primary** portion of the field, because primary radiation from all parts of the source contributes to the dose at all points in this region.

The next region is characterized by a rapid decrease in dose as you move outward from the center. This is the **penumbra** (partial shadow), where only a portion of the source is contributing primary radiation, the rest of the source being hidden by the collimation.[11,12,13] The further into the penumbra a point lies, the more the source is hidden, and thus the smaller the dose received.

The third region is characterized by a gradual decrease in dose, and has a much smaller value than in the center or penumbra. This is the **umbra** (full shadow), which receives no primary radiation except a small amount transmitted through the collimator (usually less than 1%). Most of the dose here is due to scattered radiation from primary radiation which interacts with tissue inside the field and scattering from the collimator.

Now look closely at the full primary region. You might ask why the dose is not constant throughout this region, since all points in this region receive primary radiation from all parts of the source. However, not all points receive the same amount of primary radiation, and also, the center of the region receives more scattered radiation than the edges.

There are two reasons why the amount of primary radiation differs. The first reason requires a geometrical explanation (Figure 4.10). Obviously, the distance from the source to any depth in the tissue is greater toward the edge of the field than it is at center (the hypotenuse is always the longest side of a right triangle). This difference will be more important for a short SSD, and relatively unimportant for a long SSD. In any case, the inverse square law dictates that less radiation will be received toward the edge of the field.

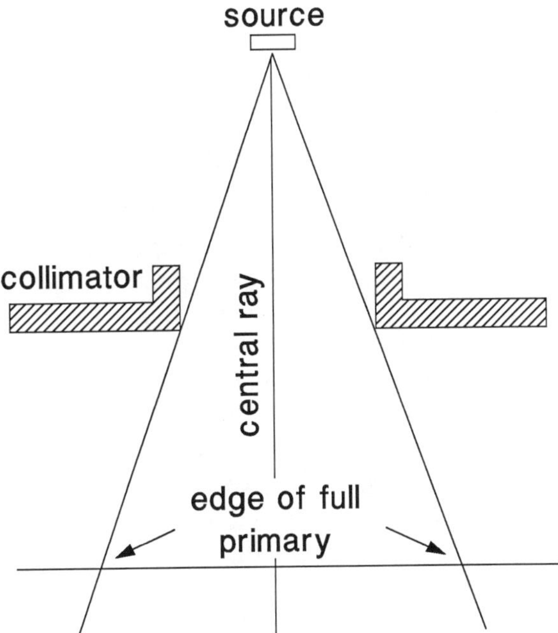

Figure 4.10 Geometrical configuration of a radiation field.

A second reason for variation in the amount of primary radiation is that x-rays do not leave the source in all directions with equal probability. This effect is more pronounced for very high energy x-rays, where the probability of x-ray production is maximized on the central ray, falling off sharply in all other directions (Figure 4.11). This is not a desirable condition. Therefore, a cone shaped beam flattening filter is placed in the beam, close to the x-ray target. Flattening filter is a poor name for this device.

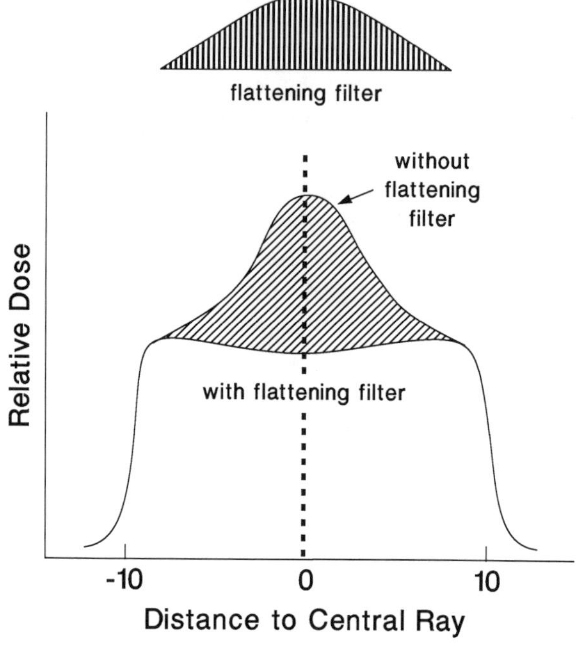

While it does necessarily do some wavelength filtering, that is not its purpose. It is really an intensity compensator. Since the filter is thickest in the center, it removes more radiation there, and less is removed toward the edges of the field. The reason for this is obvious when you look at Figure 4.11.

While it would be possible with such a filter to make the field dose profile flat at the dose maximum in the full primary region, this is not done. Instead a buildup depth dose profile like Figure 4.11 is accomplished; less dose occurs in the center, and higher dose occurs at the edges (these prominences on the dose profile are called "horns"). The reason for this design is to flatten the beam at a depth of 10 cm, a depth usually of greater clinical interest. The horns "fade away" with depth as a result of photon scattering within the tissue.

At any given depth in a field from a linear accelerator or betatron, the flattening filter has the strongest influence on the distribution of primary radiation.[14,15,16,17,18] Flattening filters are normally not used for cobalt-60 machines, since the radiation is not coming from an x-ray target, but from a radioactive source, and thus the radiation is nearly uniform at various angles in the beam.

Two kinds of scatter radiation have a profound effect on the dose profile of x-ray or gamma ray beams: collimator scatter and tissue scatter. Scatter from the collimator is a strong factor for all types of radiation. Higher energy radiation has a tendency to scatter through rather small angles (not deviating greatly from its original direction) and to retain sufficient energy after scattering to behave rather like the primary radiation. Consequently, for cobalt-60 machines, linear accelerators, and betatrons, the collimator scatter is often classed with the primary radiation in its effect on the dose profiles; i.e., whether or not the photons reach the tissue directly from the source, or deflect from the collimator, they still originate from events taking place outside the patient. Both types of photons have similar properties and capabilities when they enter the tissue. The basic difference is that collimator scattered radiation that reaches a point in the patient depends on the field size, whereas primary radiation does not.

The center of the field always receives more scattered radiation from the collimator than the edges, unless the collimator is very near or in contact with the skin, in which case the reverse may be true, particularly for low energy radiations.

Scatter from within the patient, on the other hand, will always contribute more dose to the center of the field, and less as you move away from the center. In other words, if the beam profile is flat without tissue scatter it will become rounded (become high in the center) because of tissue scatter. If the profile has "horns" initially, as in Figure 4.11, the tissue scatter will tend to level them (and eventually round off the profile at a greater depth).

With any teletherapy radiation, the importance of tissue scatter increases at greater depths, causing the dose profile to become more rounded at greater depth.

For example, of the radiation reaching a depth of 1 cm on the central axis for an 8 cm diameter from cobalt-60 at 80 cm SSD, 5% is due to scatter, and 95% is primary. At a depth of 10 cm, 25% is due to scatter, and 75% is primary. At a depth of 20 cm, 38% is due to scatter, and 62% is primary. Thus, while the amount of all types of radiation (including scatter) is less at greater depths, the importance of scatter increases.

Tissue scatter is even more important with lower energy radiation. For example, for the same 8 cm diameter field, but from intermediate (low orthovoltage) radiation with HVL of 1.0 mm copper, at 50 cm SSD, at 1 cm depth on the central axis already 48% of the radiation is due to scatter; at a 10 cm depth, 67% is due to scatter. At a 20 cm depth, virtually all of the radiation is due to scatter from the overlying tissue. For very high energy radiation, scattered radiation from the tissue plays a less important, but not a negligible, role.

Another important aspect is the change of tissue scatter with field size. Here the rule is that the larger the field, the more important is the tissue scatter. For example, for cobalt-60 at 80 cm and 15 cm depth on the central axis, for a field size of 4 x 4 cm, 17% of the radiation is due to scatter; for an 8 x 8 cm field, 28% is due to scatter; for a 12 x 12 cm field, 34% is due to scatter; and for a 20 x 20 cm field, 41% is due to scatter.

Consequently, large fields tend to have more curvature in the primary portion of the dose profiles than do small fields; low energy beams tend to have rounder profiles than high energy beams.

While a flattening filter, collimator scatter, and tissue scatter all have effects in the penumbra region, they are extremely minor in comparison to the variation in primary radiation.[11,19] To understand why this is so, consider that the amount of primary radiation reaching a point depends directly on what fraction of the source is capable of delivering radiation directly to that point; that is, what fraction of the source is not being hidden behind the collimator.

Ignore the ridiculousness of the following illustration for a moment: suppose you are an ant walking in toward the center of a radiation field - from the umbra into the penumbra and then on into the full primary field. Suppose also that you stop to look up toward the source from time to time. If no barriers (other than the collimator) are between you and the source, Figure 4.12 illustrates what you would see. (The dashed lines indicate portions of the source hidden behind the diaphragm.)

The **penumbra** is that region between the ant's stopping points 2 and 5. In this region, a part, but not all of the source is visible, so the ant (and the patient on which he walks) receives only a fraction of the primary radiation available from the source.

Obviously, if the ant continues his trek, he will pass back into the penumbra and then into the umbra on the other side of the field, repeating his experience in reverse. Thus you can see that penumbra surrounds the field.

How large is the penumbra? Consider Figure 4.13. Here the reference line is at d, a depth of interest in the patient. (If we are interested in the penumbra at the surface, we simply let d = 0 in the following.) SDD = source to diaphragm distance; DSD = diaphragm to skin distance. (Note that SDD + DSD = SSD, source to skin distance.)

Elementary geometry tells us that if we can match each of the angles in one triangle with an angle in another triangle (A=a, B=b, C=c), then the triangles are said to be **similar**, and a number of proportional relationships are true for them.

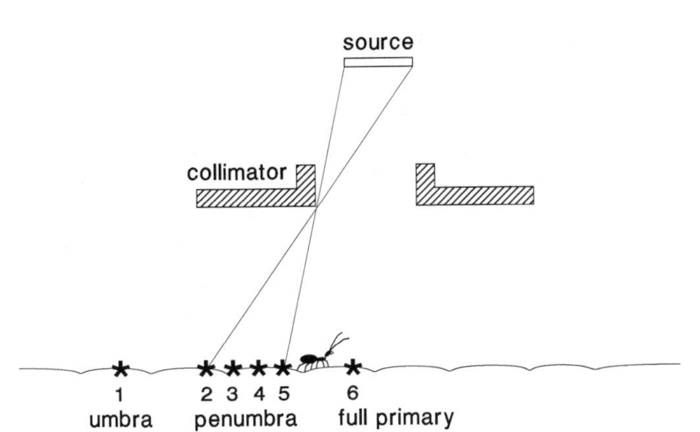

Figure 4.12. (a) Points at which the ant stops and looks up. (b) What the ant sees at the various points.

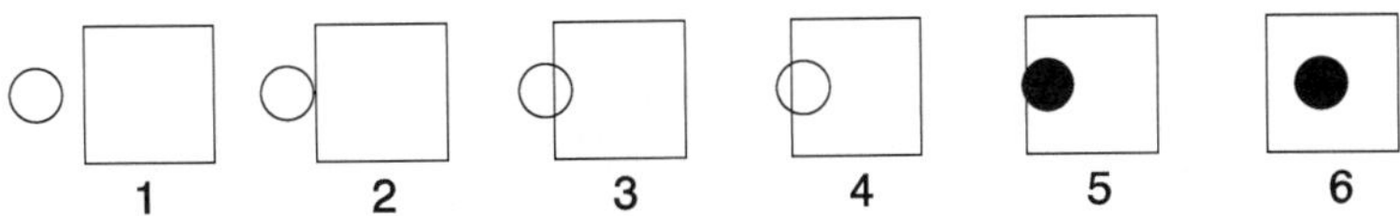

Figure 4.13

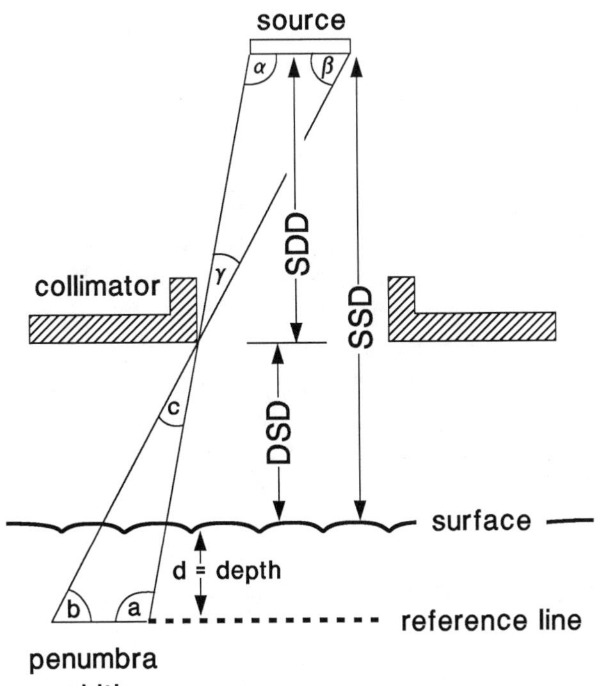

Two such triangles are those formed between point 0 and the source, with angles α, β, γ and the one formed between point 0 and the line marked "penumbra width," with angles a, b, and c. Now, angle α = angle a (a straight line intersecting parallel lines forms equal angles). Also, angle β = angle b for the same reason. Angle γ = angle c (intersecting straight lines form equal angles). Thus, the two triangles are similar.

In similar triangles, the ratio of **base** to **altitude** of one triangle equals the ratio of base to altitude for the other triangle. The base of the upper triangle is the source diameter; the base of the lower triangle is the penumbra width (P). The altitude of the upper triangle is SDD; the altitude of the lower triangle is DSD + d. Therefore:

$$\frac{penumbra\ width}{source\ diameter} = \frac{diaphragm\ skin\ distance + tissue\ depth}{source\ to\ diaphragm\ distance}$$

or:

$$P = source\ diameter \left(\frac{DSD + d}{SDD}\right)$$

For the special case of penumbra at the surface, when tissue depth is 0:

$$P = source\ diameter \left(\frac{DSD}{SDD}\right)$$

But observe that since DSD + SDD = SSD, we could write penumbra width for any depth d as:

$$P = source\ diameter \left(\frac{SSD - SDD + d}{SDD}\right)$$

From this equation, you can readily see the effect of the individual factors on the penumbra size. Obviously, if you increase the source diameter, you increase the penumbra width in direct proportion. If you increase the source-diaphragm distance, since SDD is in the denominator, the penumbra width decreases. If you increase the diaphragm skin distance (by treating at a large SSD without auxiliary blocks, for example), again the penumbra width increases in direct proportion. You might think that the ideal design would be to have an extremely small source and put the diaphragm in contact with the skin. Recall, however, that this would cause severe skin reaction, since the collimator is metal and the skin would receive much electron contamination from it.

It should be added here that small diameter cobalt sources (1 or 1.5 cm diameter) are available, but they are significantly more expensive than a 2 cm diameter source. The cobalt in the source absorbs some of the gamma rays. A smaller diameter source must be longer and thus be subject to more self absorption. Thus, obtaining a small penumbra for a telecobalt unit becomes a matter of economics.

Below are some examples of penumbra widths calculation (on the surface) for some typical equipment.

Cobalt-60. Calculate the penumbra width (P) on the surface with a source diameter of 2 cm and an SDD of 60 cm.

$$P = source\ diameter \left(\frac{SSD - SDD}{SDD} \right)$$

$$at\ 80\ cm\ SSD,\ P = 2\left(\frac{80 - 60}{60} \right) = 2\left(\frac{20}{60} \right) = 2\left(\frac{1}{3} \right) = \frac{2}{3}\ cm = 6.7\ mm$$

$$at\ 100\ cm\ SSD,\ P = 2\left(\frac{100 - 60}{60} \right) = 2\left(\frac{40}{60} \right) = 2\left(\frac{2}{3} \right) = \frac{4}{3}\ cm = 13.3\ mm$$

Clinac-4. Calculate the penumbra width on the surce with a source width (target) of 2 mm and an SDD (upper jaws) of 34 cm.

$$at\ 80\ cm\ SSD,\ P = 0.2\left(\frac{80 - 34}{34} \right) = 0.2\left(\frac{46}{34} \right) = 0.27\ cm = 2.7\ mm$$

$$at\ 100\ cm\ SSD,\ P = 0.2\left(\frac{100 - 34}{34} \right) = 0.2\left(\frac{66}{34} \right) = 3.9\ mm$$

Note that while the geometric penumbra[10,15] for the 4 MV machine is indeed small, oblique transmission of primary radiation through the collimator jaws spreads out the appearance of the penumbra so that the profile region normally considered as penumbra is about 5 mm wide at 80 cm SSD.

The equation for calculating the penumbra also tells us that the penumbra gets larger at greater depths. In fact, the penumbra grows much more rapidly than the field size does. Consider again the example of a cobalt-60 unit with an SSD of 80 cm, an SDD of 60 cm, and a source diameter of 2 cm.

$$P = source\ diameter \left(\frac{DSD + depth}{SDD} \right)\ ,where\ (DSD = SSD - SDD = 20\ cm$$

(a) at the surface, $d = 0$, therefore $P = 20\ mm = 6.7\ mm$

(b) at a depth of 10 cm, $d = 10\ cm$, therefore $P = 20\ mm\left(\frac{20\ cm + 10\ cm}{60\ cm} \right) = 10\ mm$

(c) at 20 cm depth, $d = 20\ cm$, therefore $P = 20\ mm\left(\frac{20\ cm + 20\ cm}{60\ cm} \right) = 13.3\ mm$

In going from the surface to a depth of 20 cm, the field size will increase by 25% (100 cm/80 cm = 1.25) whereas the penumbra width will increase by 100%. Obviously, the penumbra is growing more rapidly than the field.

This increase becomes more impressive when you consider the area covered by the penumbra. If the nominal field size is 10 x 10 cm and it has a 1 cm penumbra width, the actual irradiated area is 11 x 11 cm, whereas the area treated with cancer killing radiation (exclusive of penumbra), is 9 x 9 cm:

$$\text{area treated} = 11 \times 11 \ cm^2 = 121 \ cm^2$$
$$\text{area treated well} = 9 \times 9 \ cm^2 = 81 \ cm^2$$
$$\text{fraction of field "wasted"} = \frac{121 - 81}{10 \times 10} = \frac{40}{100} = 40\%$$

Thus, although the penumbra is only 10% as wide as the field in this case, it accounts for 40% as much area as the field.

It is imperative that the field size you choose to treat a target volume be large enough so that the full primary portion of the field covers the tumor. That is, all the penumbra must be outside the target area. In choosing a field, you must know how large the penumbra is at the depth of interest.

As mentioned previously, a long collimator on a cobalt-60 unit gives a relatively small penumbra (for a cobalt-60 unit). Obviously there must be a compromise, or all cobalt units would have a long collimator. The concept of isocentric treatment helps explain this compromise. With this kind of treatment, you establish the point (or line) of reference inside the patient, usually within the tumor volume, rather than on the surface. The treatment unit is designed so that the source can be rotated around this point (called the isocenter) rather like a ball on a string. This enables you to set up several fields aimed at the same target volume in a very short time with minimum setup error on all but the first field. Much more will be said about the isocentric technique later.

Imagine that we wish to treat a central volume in a pelvis measuring 34 cm laterally. If we choose to do this isocentrically at 80 cm SAD (source to axis distance), then the surface of the skin in a lateral field would be 17 cm from the isocenter, which is 63 cm from the source.

With a long collimator cobalt-60 unit, this would place the collimator virtually in contact with the skin, and an extreme skin reaction would result. Thus using a long collimator to achieve a relatively small penumbra, we give up the ability to do isocentric therapy at 80 cm SAD.

If you wish to do isocentric treatment, you should have 30 to 40 cm between the diaphragm and the isocenter. This creates a large penumbra if you are using a cobalt-60 unit which is also used for non-isocentric technique at a larger SSD.

Penumbra trimmers modify cobalt-60 units for non-isocentric techniques.[20] These are extensions which are placed on the collimator jaws and move with the jaws. When in place, they define the field edge and they can be removed for isocentric techniques. Consider, for example, a cobalt-60 unit with isocentric capability at 60 cm SAD. The normal SDD is 27.5 cm. This gives 32.5 cm between isocenter and diaphragm, permitting most isocentric techniques. But suppose you use the unit at 60 cm SSD, with a 2 cm diameter source:

$$P = 2\ cm \left(\frac{60 - 27.5}{27.5}\right) = 2.36\ cm = 23.6\ mm\ (at\ surface)$$

Obviously this is a disastrous penumbra size. Penumbra trimmers are available for this unit. They are made of depleted uranium. When in place, they extend the SDD to 45 cm, a very definite improvement:

$$P = 2\ cm \left(\frac{60 - 45}{45}\right) = 2\ cm \left(\frac{1}{4}\right) = 5\ mm\ (with\ trimmers)$$

This scheme is not used in every case because penumbra trimmers are always a compromise. Not only are they time consuming to install, but also they are necessarily (due to their delicate

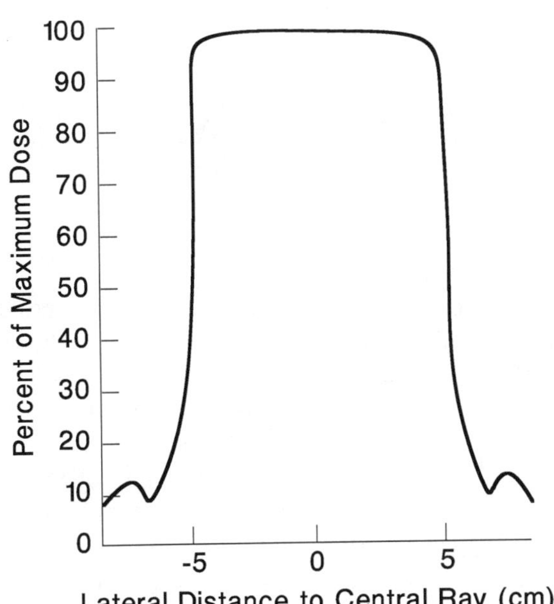

Figure 4.14. Beam profile at d_{max} for a Theratron-80 cobalt-60 unit with penumbra trimmers at 65 cm SDD. Measured with type-M film and densitometer. Note the peculiar edge effects due to the trimmers.

and lightweight construction) highly susceptible to damage which seriously affects the alignment of the light localizer field and the radiation field. Furthermore, because of their delicate nature, they can never do a fully adequate job of defining the field as can permanently mounted collimator jaws of robust construction (see Figure 4.14).

E.
Definition of Field Size

A phrase such as "a 10 x 10 cm field" can be tossed around very easily, but what does it mean? Does it mean that radiation is delivered inside a 10 x 10 cm square with no radiation outside? Obviously not, if you glance at any beam profile. Does it mean 10 x 10 cm field in full primary? What about the penumbra? Excluding the penumbra would be a suitable definition of the field, but it would be difficult to use. The light field localizer would have to vary with treatment distance since the radiation penumbra depends on the SSD. We obviously cannot see the actual radiation field, but must estimate where it is with a visible light field which simulates the radiation field (Figure 4.15).

Figure 4.15

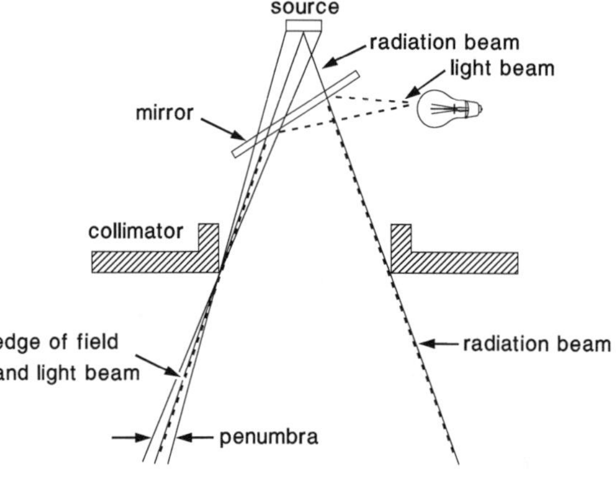

A light bulb is mounted at right angles to the source beam. Its rays are reflected off a front-silvered mirror angled to direct the light field to the collimator opening.

The reflected distance from the bulb filament to the skin must be the same as the source distance to the skin.

You will notice in Figure 4.15 that the edge of the light field (if the bulb is properly aligned and situated) falls directly in the center of the penumbra. This fact enables us to establish a sensible definition for field size which can be simulated by our light field.

Since in the center of the penumbra exactly half of the source is "visible" from the planes below the collimator, then exactly one half of the possible primary radiation will reach this line. As it turns out, approximately half as much scattered radiation also reaches this line as reaches the central ray at the same depth. Thus our definition of field size is as follows:

The edge of the radiation field is defined as the point on the major and minor axes at d_{max}, at which the dose is 50% of the dose on the central ray at the depth of maximum dose.[21]

According to this definition, the edge of the field is not exactly at the center of the penumbra. A small amount of radiation passes through the diaphragm, and slightly more than 1/2 of the scatter is present at the center of the penumbra. Thus, the 50% dose occurs just slightly outside the penumbra center. The error of about 1/2 mm or less is negligible.

The **umbra region**, outside the field, may seem the least important part to consider, since the dose here is normally 10% or less of the value in the full primary region. Nevertheless, it can be very important when critical structures, such as the lens of the eye, lie close to the field.

As noted earlier, the only radiations reaching the umbra are primary radiation transmitted through the collimator jaws, some radiation scattered by the jaw, and radiation scattered from the tissue within the field. This tissue scatter will be greater for soft radiations, and less for hard radiations. Take note of this in the upcoming comparison of isodose curves.

Isodose curves are, at present, the most clinically useful means of presenting dose information for a radiation field.[20] Imagine passing a two dimensional plane through a radiation field

Figure 4.16

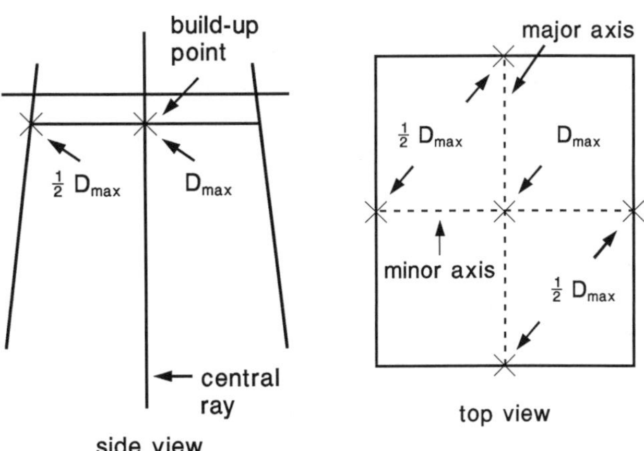

(always remember that the field is three dimensional). The most common plane for showing isodose curves is perpendicular to the surface, contains the central ray, and is oriented along the major or the minor axis of the field (Figure 4.17). Other planes of importance are off-axis but parallel to the central ray (Figure 4.18). Sometimes a plane parallel to the surface (and perpendicular to the central ray) at some specified depth is useful (Figure

Figure 4.17. Planes most often chosen for isodose display.

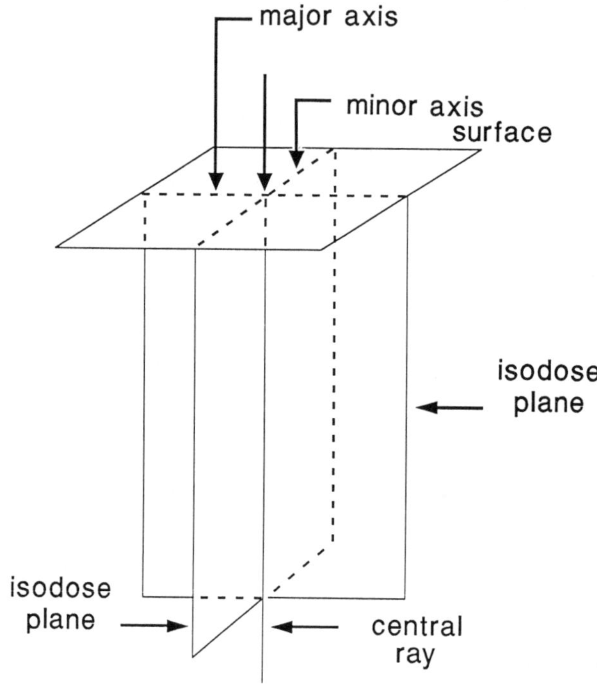

Figure 4.18. An off-axis plane for isodose display.

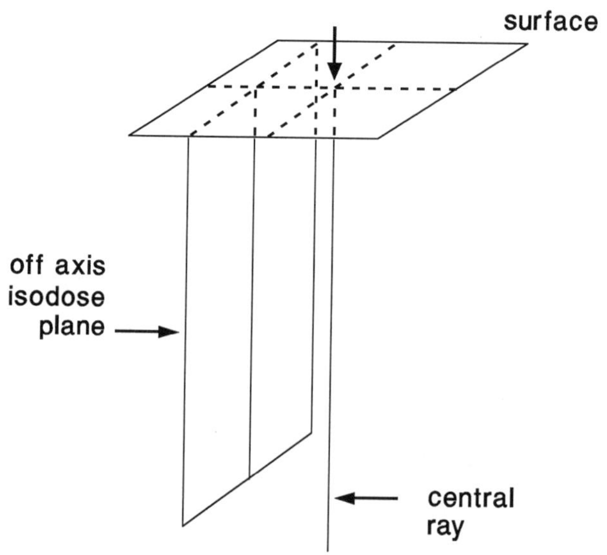

4.19). These last two representations are helpful in visualizing the three dimensional aspect of dose distribution.

Regardless of which plane is chosen, an **isodose curve** is a line connecting all points in that plane to which the same dose is given (i.e., all points on the curve are equally dosed).

The value assigned to a line in an isodose curve is normally not a quantitative dose in cGy or Gy (though it may be), but a percentage of the dose at some reference point. The reference point is normally either the point at d_{max} on the central ray or the isocenter.

Whichever reference point is chosen, it is assigned a value of 100%, and other isodose curves in the plane then take on percentage values which may be more or less than 100%.

Since dose deposition is a "smooth" and continuous phenomenon from point to point, no isodose line may begin at one point

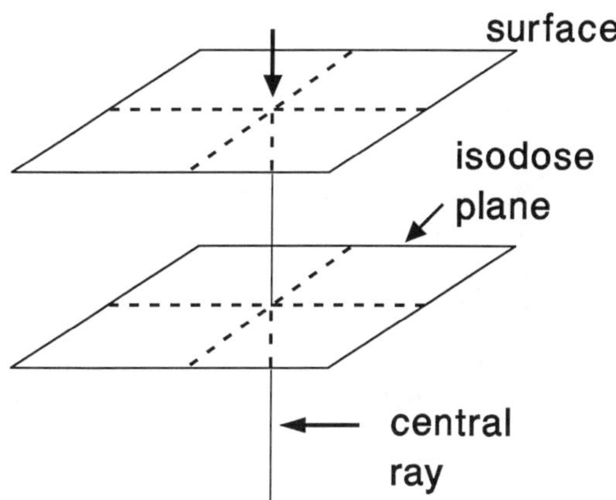

Figure 4.19. A plane for isodose display perpendicular to the central ray.

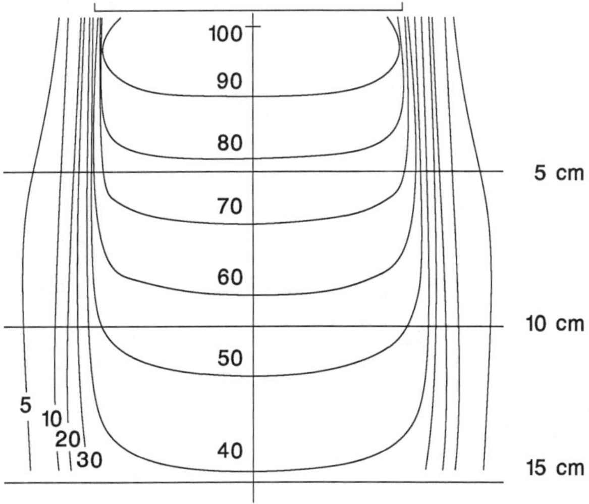

Figure 4.20. Cobalt-60, 10 x 10 cm field, 80 SSD, 60 cm SDD, 2 cm source.

within the tissue and end at a different point. They either form closed curves or begin and end at the surface.

A collection of isodose curves in a single plane is called an **isodose distribution**. It can tell you a lot about the merits of a particular beam for a cancer treatment, provided you realize you are looking at only one plane in the field.

Obviously, the depths at which the isodose lines cross the central ray (if they do) must agree with the data from depth dose curves or tables for that treatment machine.

Figure 4.20 is a typical isodose distribution for a plane similar to those in Figure 4.17. The field is a 10 x 10 cm cobalt-60 field at 80 cm SSD, with perpendicular entry into a flat surface.

Note the full primary region of the field. Near the surface, the lines are relatively flat, though they have a slight upward curvature as you move away from central ray (indicating that the dose is decreasing slightly in this direction). As you go deeper, the lines become more rounded (the effect of increased scatter radiation).

In the penumbra region the lines are close together (indicating a very rapid change in dose from point to point) and are more nearly vertical (more nearly parallel to the edge of the field). Also note that the penumbra gets wider at greater depth (the isodose lines become less crowded).[12]

In the umbra region there are few lines, since there is little dose in this region, and the dose does not change rapidly from point to point as in the penumbra. Notice the slight bulging of the 5% dose at the bottom, an effect of the buildup of lateral scatter with depth.

Note that the distance between 50% isodose curves on the two sides at the depth of d_{max} (5 mm) is slightly more than the nominal field width, 10 cm (which was determined by a light localizer field).

References

1. Attix, F.H. *Introduction to Radiological Physics and Radiation Dosimetry*, John Wiley & Sons, New York, 1986, Chapter 4.
2. Meredith, W.J. & Massey, J.B. *Fundamental Physics of Radiology*, 3rd Edition, John Wright & Sons, Bristol, Great Britain, 1976, pp. 449-451.
3. Johns, H.E. & Cunningham, J.R. *The Physics of Radiology*, 4th Edition, Charles C. Thomas, Springfield, 1983, pp. 220-223.

4. *Determination of Absorbed Dose in a Patient Irradiated by Beams of X or Gamma Rays in Radiotherapy*, Report 24, International Commission on Radiation Units, Washington, D.C., 1976, p. 52.

5. Ibid., p. 55.

6. Burkell, C.C., Watson, T.A., Johns, H.E., Horsley, R.J. "Skin Effects of Cobalt 60 Telecurie Therapy," *Br J Radiol* 27:171, 1954.

7. White, D.R. "Tissue Substitute in Experimental Radiation Physics," *Med Phys* 5:467, 1978.

8. Ibbott, G. & Hendee, W. "Beam-Shaping Platforms and Skin-Sparing Advantage of Cobalt 60 Radiation, *Am J Roentgenol* 108:193, 1970.

9. Johns, H.E., Epp, E.R., Cormack, D.V., Fedoruk, S.O. "Depth Dose Data and Diaphragm Design for Saskatchewan 1,000 Curie Cobalt Unit," *Br J Radiol* 25:302, 1952.

10. Podgorsak, E.B., Rawlison, J.A., Johns, H.E. "X-Ray Depth Doses from Linear Accelerators in the Energy Range from 10 to 32 MeV," *Am J Roentgenol* 123:182, 1975.

11. ICRU Report 24, pp. 12, 37, 54.

12. Johns & Cunningham, pp. 105, 119, 370.

13. Debois, J. "The Determination of the Penumbra at Different Depths," *J Belge Radiol* 49:200, 1966.

14. Kerst, D.W. "The Betatron," *Radiology*, 40:115, 1943.

15. Johns & Cunningham, p. 106.

16. Adams, G.D. et al. "Techniques for Application of the Betatron to Medical Therapy," *Am J Roentgenol* 60:153, 1948.

17. Johns, H.E., Darby, E.K., Haslam, R.N.H., Katz, L., Harrington, E.L. "Depth Dose Data and Isodose Distributions for Radiation From a 22 MeV Betatron," *Amer J Roentgen* 62:257, 1949.

18. Skaggs, L.S., Almy, D.M., Kerst, D.W., Lanzl, L.H. "Development of Betatron for Electron Therapy, With Introduction on the Therapeutic Principles of Fast Electrons," *Radiology* 50:167, 1948.

19. Khan, F.M. *The Physics of Radiation Therapy*, Williams & Wilkins, Baltimore, 1984, pp. 63-65.

20. Ibid., p. 65.

21. ICRU Report 24, p. 53.

Characteristics of Electron Beams

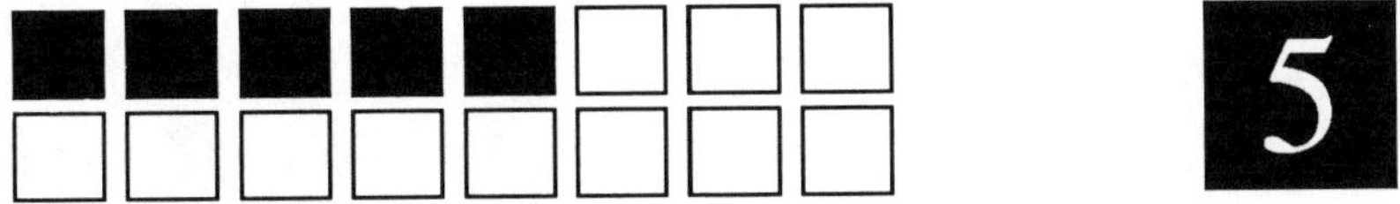

5

A. *Electron Range*
B. *Skin Dose and Dose Buildup for Electron Beams*
C. *Normalization Depth*
D. *Electron Beam Depth Dose Curves*
E. *Electron Beam Isodose Curves*
F. *The Importance of Diaphragm to Skin Distance*
G. *The Effect of Tissue Inhomogeneities*

A.
Electron Range

There is one major difference between the absorption of electrons and photons. When a beam of photons enters an absorbing medium, the photons penetrate to all depths within the medium. Although the number of photons is constantly reduced as the beam penetrates deeper, the beam is still there, regardless of the depth. Electrons, on the other hand, penetrate only to a certain depth (depending on the initial electron energy) but no deeper; i.e., electrons have a definite maximum range, whereas photons do not. For example, the range for 18 MeV electrons is 9 cm in water. This means that all electrons will stop by 9 cm depth, but none will reach 9.5 cm. The advantage of using electron beams is obvious when you consider a diseased volume at a depth o f 5 cm with a sensitive healthy tissue directly under it at 10 cm depth.

An empirical formula (empirical means it cannot be derived from valid physical principles, but just happens to work by coincidence) for the range (R) of electrons having energies useful in teletherapy is:

$$R\ (cm) = 0.521\ E_0\ (MeV) - 0.376$$

where R is the range in cm of water or muscle and E_0 is the initial energy of the electrons in MeV before they enter the water or muscle.[1,2,3]

Using this equation, ranges for various electron energies are given in Table 5.1.

Table 5.1

Initial Energy (MeV)	4	6	9	12	15	18	24
Range in water (cm)	1.7	2.75	4.3	5.9	7.4	9.0	12.1

Rather than remembering the formula, you may use the rough approximation, which can be seen from the above. The range (cm) of electrons in tissue is roughly half the energy in MeV. The range is actually somewhat less for energies below 18 MeV, and more for energies above 18 MeV.

Although the actual range is given by the formula above, the useful range for cancer therapy is considerably less. The depth dose and isodose curves show that the dose for electron beams falls rapidly at depths beyond the 80 percent isodose line. For this reason, it is customary to select an electron energy beam in which the target (cancer) volume is completely encompassed by the 85 percent isodose curve. The approximate depths at which this dose lies for the Varian Clinac-18 are given in Table 5.2.

Another rough approximation for electron beams is that the useful therapy range is about half of the maximum range, or about 1/4 of the energy in MeV.

Table 5.2

Initial Energy (MeV)	6	9	12	15	18
Range (cm)	2.75	4.3	5.9	7.4	9.0
Depth of 85% line (cm)	1.4	2.4	3.3	4.3	5.0

B.
Skin Dose and Dose Buildup for Electron Beams

There is a skin sparing effect with electron beams, but in general it is not as great as with photon beams. Quantitatively, the effect depends on the energy, the field size, and the method used to produce beam spreading.

Beam spreading is necessary because the electron beam emerging from the machine is usually very narrow (like a thick pencil lead), which of course would provide an inadequate treatment area. Spreading is normally, but not always, accomplished by placing **scattering foils** into the beam between the accelerator window and the collimator.[4] The larger the field and/or the higher the electron energy, the thicker the scattering foil needed. The scattering foil has a rather large effect on three important factors: the percent skin dose, the buildup depth, and the useful therapy range (the position of the 80% isodose line).

With higher energies and larger fields, the percent skin dose is higher, buildup occurs more quickly, and the relative useful therapy range is increased. Quantitatively, the skin dose for a small field at 6 MeV may be about 70% of the maximum dose, while for a large field at the same energy it may be 80%. For 18 MeV electrons, these doses would be about 85% for a small (4 x 4 cm) field and nearly 100% for a large (20 x 20 cm) field.

The depth at which maximum dose (d_{max}) occurs also depends on energy, but not in a straightforward manner. For example, at 6 MeV, d_{max} occurs at approximately 10 mm; for 9 MeV, d_{max} is at about 15 mm; and for 12 MeV, d_{max} occurs at about 19 mm. Thus you see a trend of greater d_{max} at higher energy. At 15 MeV, however, d_{max} may occur at about 10 mm, depending on field size. This reversal is due to the effect of the scattering foil, which spreads the energy of the beam before it reaches the tissue.

C.
Normalization Depth

As mentioned earlier, it is customary to express the dose in an irradiated medium as a percentage (or fraction) of the dose at some reference point which is assigned a value of 100% or 1.0. When this is done, the dose is said to be **normalized** at this reference point, and the depth of the reference point in the medium is called the **normalization depth.**

For photon teletherapy, the normalization point is usually either at the point of maximum dose on the central ray, or at the isocenter. Since electron beams are not used isocentrically, it would seem logical to normalize at the maximum point. As was pointed out above, however, the depth of maximum dose for electron beams depends on a great many factors, including field size and energy. Thus if you were to normalize at the maximum point, the normalization depth would be at a great many different depths - a highly confusing situation and a great time-consuming inconvenience when the outputs are being calibrated.

For these reasons, the normalization depths are chosen as listed in Table 5.3.

Table 5.3

Initial Energy (MeV)	2 - 4.99	5 - 9.99	10 -19.99	20 - 50
Normalization Depth (cm)	0.5	1.0	2.0	3.0

The normalization depth does not often coincide with the depth of maximum dose, and for higher energies may not even be within a centimeter of it; but it is always at a point whose dose is close to maximum. Thus it is possible to have depth dose percentages greater than 100%, but rarely in excess of 103%.

D.

Electron Beam Depth Dose Curves

Figures 5.1 through 5.3 are examples of depth dose curves which demonstrate some of the aspects of electron beams discussed thus far. Observe, for example, variation in skin dose and d_{max} with field size and energy, and the rapid decrease in dose after the 80% depth dose.

Another interesting feature of these curves is that the dose does not fall to zero. Rather, dose decreases rapidly to a point near the maximum range, levels off to a value of a few percent and then decreases very slowly.

It was stated earlier that electrons do not contribute to dose beyond their range. How then can you explain this "tailing off" phenomenon? The answer is that the dose in this tail region is not due to electrons coming from the accelerator, but is due rather to x-rays produced by the electron beam. These x-rays are

Figure 5.1,
Figure 5.2

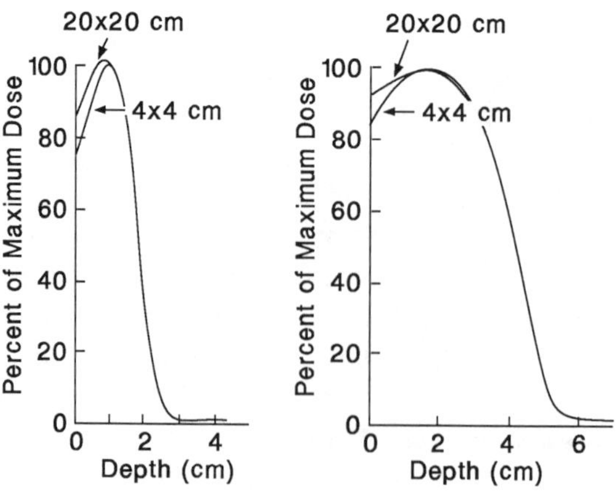

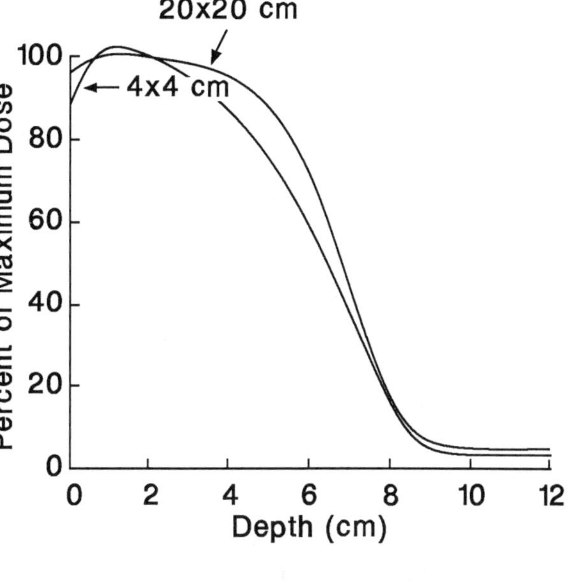

Figure 5.3

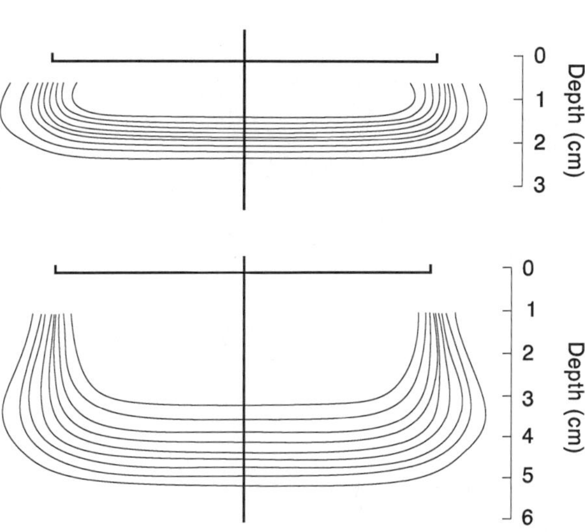

Figure 5.4

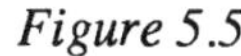

Figure 5.5

Figure 5.6

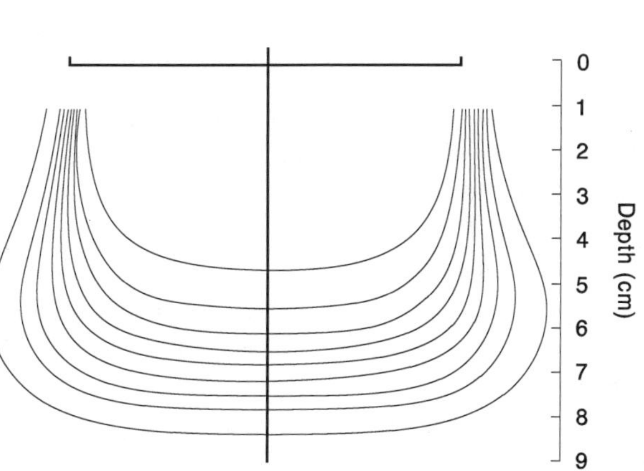

bremsstrahlung radiation, the same as most of the x-rays coming from a conventional x-ray tube. The bremsstrahlung phenomenon occurs whenever fast moving electrons interact with matter.[5,6,7] The higher the atomic number of the matter and the higher the energy of the electrons, the more bremsstrahlung is produced.[8]

Two factors affect bremsstrahlung production: (a) the tissue of the patient and (b) the metal of the scattering foil and the collimator. Nothing can be done about the bremsstrahlung coming from the patient. Tissue with its low atomic number produces little bremsstrahlung. However, the bremsstrahlung from the collimator is reduced if the collimator is made of a low atomic number material such as aluminum.

Note also that if you extrapolate the curves of figures 5.1, 5.2, and 5.3, the depth at which the electron curves would reach zero dose in the absence of bremsstrahlung does not correspond to the range of electrons at these energies (see Table 5.1), but is somewhat less. This is because the nominal energies listed are not the true electron energies as they reach the patient, but the approximate energies of electrons at the end of the accelerator section of the machine. The energy is reduced beyond this point by the exit window, the scattering foil, and the dose measuring system before the electrons reach the patient.

E.

Electron Beam Depth Dose Curves

A two dimensional view of these phenomena can be seen in figures 5.4 through 5.6. You can see some additional important phenomena concerning dose at the edge of the field.

First, note the bulging of the isodose distributions toward the bottom. This is a result of electron scattering as the electrons penetrate and lose energy. Obviously it is a feature which must be kept in mind when treating with electrons, particularly when adjacent fields are used.

Note also the difference in the rate at which dose decreases at the edge of the field for low energy versus high energy electrons. (This is indicated by the spacing of the isodose lines.) The dose falls off somewhat more gradually for low energy electrons, a result of beam spreading at the end of the collimation. This is more pronounced for low energy electrons because they are more easily deflected. This is of obvious importance in deciding upon the field size for a given target volume.

Compare the "flatness" of the 80% and 90% isodose curves for low energy versus high energy electrons. Note that the curvature, indicating a decrease in dose away from the central ray, becomes more pronounced for higher energy beams.

All of the above phenomena are vital in optimum planning for treatment with electron beams and all require an assessment of isodose distributions, since the phenomena cannot be demonstrated by simple depth dose tables. The importance of consulting isodose distributions when using even single fields should be obvious.

F.

The Importance of Diaphragm to Skin Distance

As mentioned above, the end of the collimation causes beam spreading due to electron scatter, which in turn is responsible for the dose decreasing more gradually at the edge of the field. This phenomenon corresponds to penumbra in the case of x-rays, as in that case, it can lead to undertreatment of cancer tissue if it is close to the edge of the field.

This analogy to penumbra extends to the nature of the factors which control the size of the region in question. The most important of these factors (in fact, the only one which can be easily controlled) is the diaphragm to skin distance (DSD).

The greater the DSD, the less sharp the edge of the field will be.

In some treatment machines, the diaphragm is a cone which is brought into contact with the skin. Electron cones allow the insertion of a standard or customized block at their ends; this allows a variety of field shapes and sizes, but does not change the DSD. While this minimizes the penumbra effect, it obviously limits the field sizes to the number of cones on hand. Some 18 MeV machines use a series of adjustable diaphragms which are positioned 5 cm from the skin. When a large field is used on a sloping skin surface, however, at least one side of the field will be more than 5 cm away. Often nothing is done to compensate for this greater penumbra, but sometimes it is wise to lay lead strips on the skin (the analog of penumbra trimmers). In any case, you should be aware of the consequences of a large DSD.

G.
The Effect of Tissue Inhomogeneities

Depth dose and isodose information assumes a uniform water medium. The change in the isodose data due to the presence of inhomogeneities such as bone or air can be calculated, provided you know the density of the material. Unfortunately, the density of bone varies from about 1.3 to 1.8 gram per cubic centimeter, depending on its type and location.

The **equivalent depth method** is the most used method for calculating the effect of inhomogeneities on dose distribution. To use this, you must first determine the equivalent thickness of unit density tissue for the inhomogeneity; i.e., that thickness of muscle which will be affected by the beam as the actual thickness of the inhomogeneity. Since electrons interact in the tissue by collision with electrons already present in the tissue, it can be said that if a medium has the same number of electrons per cubic centimeter (electron density) as muscle, it is equivalent to muscle (one to one equivalence in thickness). If a material has twice as many electrons per cm^3 as muscle, then a given thickness of that material is equivalent to twice that thickness of muscle, and so on. In general:

$$Equivalent\ muscle\ thickness = thickness\ of\ medium \cdot \frac{(\#\ electrons/cm^3)_{medium}}{(\#\ electrons/cm^3)_{muscle}}$$

The number of electrons per cm^3 of a material depends on the number of $gram/cm^3$ (the mass density) as follows:

$$\frac{\#\ electrons}{cm^3} = \frac{\#\ electrons}{gram} \cdot \frac{\#\ grams}{cm^3}$$

Some important values for the number of electrons per gram for different medium are: muscle, 3.31×10^{23}; air, 3.34×10^{23}; bone, 3.19×10^{23}; and fat, 3.37×10^{23}.

Example 5.1:

Find the muscle equivalent thickness of 1.5 cm of bone, if the density of the bone is 1.6 $gram/cm^3$.

$$Electron\ density\ of\ muscle = \frac{\#\ electrons}{gram\ of\ muscle} \cdot \frac{\#\ grams}{cm^3\ of\ muscle}$$

$$= 3.31 \times 10^{23} \times 1.0 \frac{electrons}{cm^3}$$

$$= 3.31 \times 10^{23}\ electrons\ per\ cm^3$$

$$Electron\ density\ of\ bone = 3.19\ x\ 10^{23}\frac{electrons}{grams}\ x\ 1.6\frac{grams}{cm^3}$$

$$= 5.10\ x\ 10^{23}\ electrons\ /\ cm^3$$

$$Equivalent\ muscle\ thickness = 1.5\,cm\ \frac{5.10\ x\ 10^{23}}{3.31\ x\ 10^{23}} = 2.31\ cm$$

Assume the mass density of muscle to be 1.0 gram/cm^3. Having found the equivalent muscle thickness, you can calculate the difference between the thickness of the bone inhomogeneity and the equivalent muscle thickness. You add this difference to the depth of the point at which you wish to estimate the dose, and then proceed to use a standard depth dose curve. For instance, in the above example, the thickness difference is 2.31 cm - 1.5 cm = 0.8 cm. Thus, if you were interested in the dose to a point at a depth of 4 cm, and 1.5 cm of bone (density = 1.6 gram/cm^3) lies between the surface and this point, you would estimate the equivalent depth to be 4.8 cm rather than 4.0 cm, and find the dose percent on the appropriate depth dose curve for that energy and field size.

References

1. Markus, B. "Energiebestimmung Schneller Elektronen aus Tiefendasiskurven," *Strahlentherapic* 116:280, 1961.

2. Markus, B. "Beitrage zur Entwicklung der Dosimetrie Schneller Elektronen," *Strahlentherapie* 123:350, 508 and 124:33, 1964.

3. Katz, L. & Penfold, A.S. "Range-Energy Relations for Electrons and the Determination of Beta-Ray Endpoint Energies by Absorption," *Rev Mod Phys*, 24:28, 1951.

4. *The Use of Electron Linear Accelerators in Medical Radiation Therapy: Physical Characteristics*, U.S. Department of Health, Education, and Welfare, Bureau of Radiological Health, Rockville, 1976, p. 18.

5. Widner, R.T. & Sells, R.L. *Elementary Modern Physics*, 2nd Edition, 1976, p. 115.

6. Johns, H.E. & Cunningham, J.R. *The Physics of Radiology*, 4th Edition, Charles C. Thomas, Springfield, 1983, pp. 61, 195, 218.

7. Khan, F. *The Physics of Radiation Therapy*, Williams & Wilkins, Baltimore, 1984, p. 41.

8. Hendee, W.R. *Medical Radiation Physics, Roentgenology, Nuclear Medicine, and Ultrasound*, 2nd Edition, Year Book Medical Publishers, Chicago, 1979, p. 46.

Interpreting Machine Data Tables

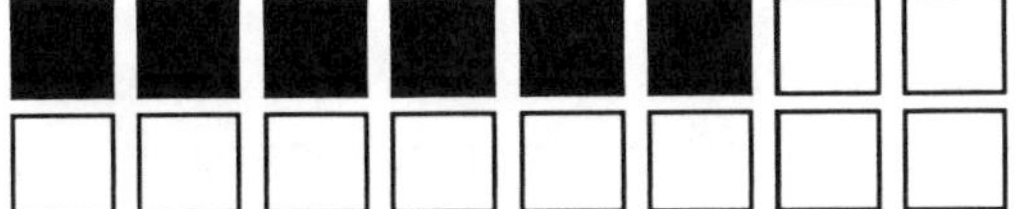 

A. *Miniphantoms and Maxiphantoms*
B. *Dose Rate Measurements versus Integrated Dose Measurements*
C. *Exposure (or Exposure Rate) in Air*
D. *Dose (or Dose Rate) in a Miniphantom*
E. *Dose (or Dose Rate) in a Maxiphantom*
F. *AAPM Protocol Calibration Techniques*
G. *Parameters on the Machine Data Tables*
H. *Monitor Factors and Field Size Dependence Factors*

Each radiation treatment unit should have a set of tables giving output and other dosimetry parameters under various clinically relevant conditions. These tables are prepared by a medical physicist, from machine calibrations and other measurements. They are used by dosimetrists, radiotherapists, physicists, etc., in calculating patient doses.

It is not the purpose of this chapter to teach you how to do machine calibrations. However, in order to use the tables correctly, you must know what the various labels and parameters mean. If you misinterpret the data, a sizeable error can occur in treatment planning.

Before you use any machine data tables, you should be sure that you know exactly what the numbers represent. There are several ways in which the machine can be calibrated, and even more ways to present the data. It sometimes happens that not all pertinent information is included in the tables. If this happens, do not make assumptions, but obtain the facts from the person who performed the calibrations.

A.
Miniphantoms and Maxiphantoms

A **phantom** is an inanimate object or extended medium within which radiation measurements are performed. It may resemble in shape a portion or all of a patient, a large or small simple box, or may merely be a small sphere or cylinder of buildup material. Whatever the shape, all phantoms should have one characteristic in common: the material should be as nearly tissue equivalent as is practical. This means that the phantom should absorb radiation just as the tissue would. This condition will hold true if the mass density, number of electrons per gram, and effective atomic numbers are the same for the two materials. For higher energy radiations, the matching of atomic numbers is not as important as matching the other two properties.

Two types of standard phantoms are worthy of special note not only because they appear in the definitions of several dosimetry parameters (TMR, TAR, TPR, and depth dose percent, which will be discussed in Chapter 8), but also because they are used for routine calibration procedures.

A **miniphantom** is a sphere of tissue equivalent medium surrounding a point of interest (or a constant thickness around the air volume of a measuring chamber) of just sufficient size to provide buildup at the center (or at the edge of the air volume of the chamber). A measurement in a miniphantom may also be referred to as being "in air" or "with buildup cap." Many ionization chambers come with cobalt-60 buildup caps (plastic 0.5 cm thick) which are thus miniphantoms for cobalt-60 beams.

A **maxiphantom** is an extended phantom large enough so that if it were larger it would make no difference in the dose to any point of interest. A maxiphantom is sometimes called a "semi-infinite" phantom, but this is a contradiction in terms.

To understand the importance of a sufficiently large maxiphantom, consider the following experiment. You construct a medium sized rectangular box, fill it with water, and then insert a waterproofed ion chamber into the water and expose it to a radiation beam. You will record a particular dose rate. If you then add some phantom material beyond the chamber, and to the sides, and make the same exposure, you will obtain a reading higher than the first. The reason is that, in the second case, you expose your chamber to all of the primary and scattered radiation present for the first reading, plus some additional backscattered and sidescattered radiation from the added phantom material.

You continue this process of adding more material until you find no increase in dose rate. The reason there is no further increase in dose rate is because, although additional scattered radiation occurred in the most recently added material, it is so far from the probe that it does not return to the probe to contribute to the dose at that point. No matter how much more phantom material is added at the end or to the sides of the existing phantom beyond this point, no difference will be observed between consecutive readings because of this addition. Your phantom is now a maxiphantom.

The amount of material which needs to be added to the bottom and sides is generally 10 to 15 cm, depending on the energy of the photon radiation; it would be considerably less for electrons.

B.
Dose Rate Measurements versus Integrated Dose Measurements

In teleisotope units (such as cobalt-60), radiation results from the disintegration of radioactive atoms, a highly predictable phenomenon. Thus the exposure rate or dose rate at a fixed point will not vary during the treatment except at the beginning or end of the treatment, when the source itself is in motion. For this reason, it is adequate to calibrate such a unit in terms of dose rate or exposure rate, and make a small correction for these end effects, called a **shutter or timer correction.**[1,2] (Usually a few seconds is added to or subtracted from the calculated treatment time).*

Another way to calibrate is to install an integrating dosimeter directly into the treatment unit and have it terminate the exposure when a pre-set dose has been delivered. This integrating dosimeter in turn should be compared frequently to measurements with a secondary dosimeter whose accuracy is traceable to the National Bureau of Standards.

The second method is somewhat more expensive, but it corrects for fluctuations in exposure rate during the treatment. Since teleisotope units do not suffer such fluctuations, the first and cheaper method is normally employed. Bear in mind that both methods work for teleisotope units.

High energy x-ray units (such as linear accelerators) utilize several complex electrical circuits to produce radiation. If there are fluctuations in any one of several electrical parameters during treatment (and there invariably are), then the rate at which radiation is produced will change. If the integrating dosimeter is used, however, the instantaneous rate becomes relatively unimportant; so long as the proper total dose is delivered, it matters little whether it took 60 seconds or 65 seconds. Thus it is necessary to use the integrating dosimeter with high energy x-ray units.

Superficial x-ray generators do not use integrating dosimeters. Recall that superficial x-rays are very "soft," so that most

---

* dose = dose rate · (timer setting ± timer correction).

of the absorption takes place within a small depth. If an integrating monitor were built into such a unit, the beam would be hardened by filtration from the ion chamber,[3,4,5] thus partially defeating the purpose of the x-ray unit. For this reason, even though the exposure rate from a superficial unit fluctuates slightly because of its electrical origin, calibration is normally in terms of exposure rate or dose rate rather than integrated dose. As a result, the dose from such a unit can never be very precise.

C.
Exposure (or Exposure Rate) in Air

This type of calibration is performed in a miniphantom and the results are expressed in roentgens per minute (rate calibration) or roentgens per monitor unit (integrator calibration). This number must be multiplied by the f-factor discussed in Chapter 1 in order to convert to dose in Gy, and by a backscatter factor to be discussed later.

While it is possible to calibrate in this fashion for any radiation with photon energies up to 3 MeV, the only cases where this is justified is for superficial and softer radiations.

D.
Dose (or Dose Rate) in a Miniphantom

Dose rate in a miniphantom differs from the exposure rate in air in that you need not multiply by an f-factor. You must still multiply either by a backscatter factor, a peak scatter factor, or a tissue-air ratio, to get the dose in a maxiphantom or a patient. It may be that the actual measurements are the same, and the calibrator merely multiplied by an f-factor before recording the results on the output sheet, or the calibrator may not have been able to measure an exposure rate (i.e., if the radiation consists of particles, such as electrons, or if it consists of photons having energies greater than 3 MeV).

An output expression such as this is directly suited for use with tissue-air ratios (TAR), to be discussed in Chapter 8.

E.
Dose (or Dose Rate) in a Maxiphantom

Determining dose rate in a maxiphantom may be done in either of two ways, although the second way is highly recommended.
(a) The chamber is placed at the depth of maximum dose (d_{max})

in a maxiphantom, and Gy per minute or Gy per monitor unit are measured.

(b) The chamber is placed at some depth other than at d_{max}, and the monitor unit or the dose rate is calibrated.

When calibrating in this manner, it is not necessary to use either an f-factor or a backscatter factor. Such measurements are directly suited for use with depth dose fractions (percent depth dose), tissue-maximum ratios (TMR), or tissue-phantom ratios (TPR), to be discussed in Chapter 8.

F.
AAPM Protocol Calibration Techniques

The protocol from the American Association of Physicists in Medicine (AAPM), contained in Report TG-21[6] and ICRU 14,[7] recommends that the calibration of photon and electron beams be performed as follows:

(a) X-rays up to 150 kVp: exposure or exposure rate measured in air.

(b) X-rays from 2 MV to 10 MV, teleisotope sources (cesium-137, cobalt-60): dose or dose rate in a maxiphantom at a depth of 5 cm.

(c) X-rays from 11 MV to 25 MV: dose or dose rate in a maxiphantom at a depth of 7 cm.

(d) X-rays from 26 MV to 50 MV: dose or dose rate in a maxiphantom at a depth of 10 cm.

In each of the above cases, the numbers on the calibration sheet may represent dose at the calibration depth or may have been converted to dose at d_{max} by dividing the depth dose fraction from tables set up for that treatment unit.

There are several reasons for calibrating according to this method. The maxiphantom is preferred because all backscatter is included in the measurement, and neither artificially introduced backscatter factors nor an f-factor is required since the calibration is in grays (with the exception of low energy x-rays).

More importantly, the reason for using the depths specified is as follows: suppose the depth dose tables you are using are in error by 4% at a depth of 10 centimeters. This is not a remarkable error, since many departments use "standard" depth dose tables, measured elsewhere for a similar machine. No two treatment units are exactly alike. This is especially true for x-ray machines and linacs, but it is true even for cobalt-60 units.

Figure 6.1 shows the situation as outlined. Even though the error in using standard tables is 4% at 10 cm depth, the error at

d_{max} is essentially zero, since the data are normalized there (this is assuming the calibration was performed at d_{max}). Assume further that the error at 5 cm depth is 2%.

Now suppose that the calibration is performed at a depth of 5 cm instead of at d_{max}. The situation would then be as pictured in Figure 6.2.

There is now no error at 5 cm depth (at least no error due to using standard depth dose curves), and only a 2% error at 10 cm, whereas a 2% error has been introduced at d_{max}. The error introduced at d_{max} is a good trade off for the reduction of error in the depth range from 5 to 10 cm, usually the most clinically significant region.

Figure 6.1

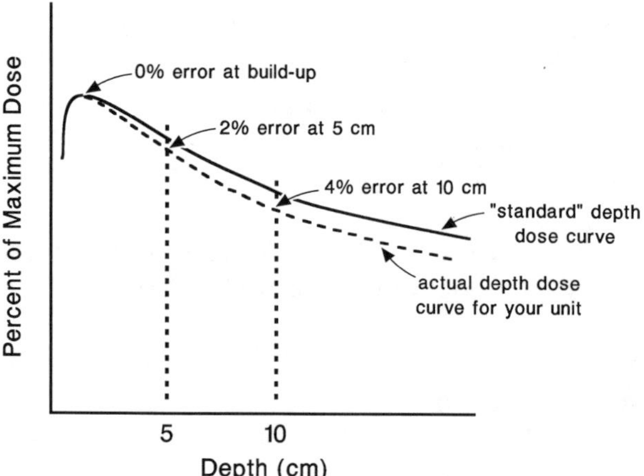

Figure 6.2

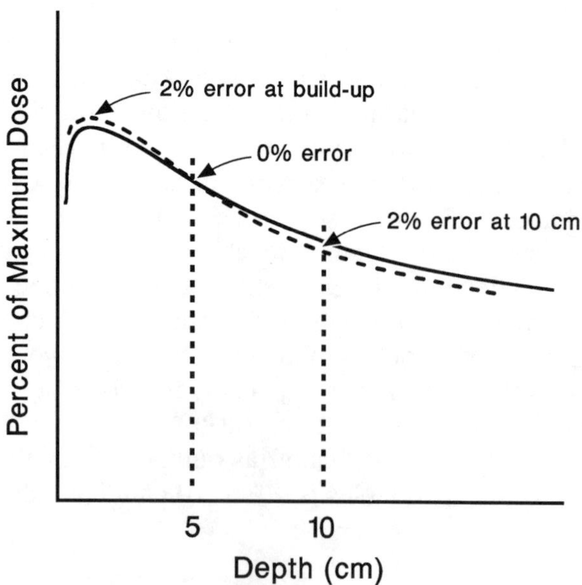

G.
Parameters on the Machine Data Tables

Before using the machine data tables, you should check certain qualifiers or parameters to be sure they match the situation for which you plan to use it. In particular, check:

(a) Correct treatment unit. Obviously a gross error will occur if you use a calibration sheet from a Clinac-18 to do orthovoltage treatment planning.

(b) Date. This is most important in the case of teleisotope units, where radioactive decay can significantly change the output over a few months, but may also be a factor for linacs, since electrical parameters can change, parts must be replaced, etc.

(c) Distance (SSD, SAD). This parameter has one obvious and one subtle aspect. An obvious error is that if the sheet says the calibration is valid at 80 cm, and your patient is positioned at 85 cm, you are making a 13% error unless you make the proper inverse square law correction.

A more subtle error is frequently made. Suppose the calibration is valid at 80 cm from the source for an 80 cm SAD unit. If you use these data for isocentric planning, no error is involved since the normalization point is at the isocenter, 80 cm from the source. If you are doing non-isocentric SSD treatment, however, then you will be using depth dose tables, normalized at buildup, and the buildup point is not at 80 cm, unless buildup occurs on the skin.

For example, when positioning a patient at 80 cm SSD on a Clinac-4, the buildup (normalization) point is 81 cm from the source, while the monitor factor is correct at 80 cm. The error will be:

$$\left(\frac{81}{80}\right)^2 - 1 = 0.025, \text{ or } 2\tfrac{1}{2}\%$$

unless the correction is made in treatment planning. This is a correction which is easy to neglect. For this reason, when treating a patient using SSD techniques on Clinac-4, the distance correction must be made when calculating treatment duration, or when the correct position is entered into the treatment planning computer. An alternative approach is to use 79 cm SSD rather than 80 cm, so that the normalization point and calibration point coincide for either SSD or SAD techniques, and a correction is not necessary.

(d) Field size. There is a variation in output not only with field size, but also with field shape, due to varying conditions of photon scatter both in the patient and from the collimation.

This variation is not purely a function of area of the field, but of both area and elongation (departure from squareness). Obviously, if you were to express an output for each useable rectangular field, the output sheet would be large and clumsy. It is customary to reduce a rectangular field to an equivalent square field for purposes of finding output, TMR (defined in Chapter 8) depth dose, backscatter, etc.

Consider two fields, one having dimensions 5 x 20 cm, the other 10 x 10 cm. Both have an area of 100 cm^2, but measurement would show that patient scatter and collimator scatter would be greater for the square field. In fact, detailed measurements would show that the 5 x 20 cm field is equivalent in output, depth dose, etc., to a square field whose dimensions are only 8 x 8 cm (see the following example).

How then are you to know the equivalent square for a rectangular field? There are tables for equivalent squares in various references.[8] However, a simple approximation is that the length of the side of the equivalent square is the area of the field divided by the average edge length. If the rectangle has dimensions A and B:

$$area = AB, \ average \ side = \frac{(A + B)}{2}$$

So:

$$Equivalent \ square \ side = \frac{2AB}{A + B}$$

For the above example (5 x 20 cm field), the equivalent square side is:

$$Equivalent \ square \ side = \frac{2AB}{A + B} = \frac{2 \times 5 \times 20}{5 + 20} = \frac{200}{25} = 8 \ cm$$

This scheme works well for fields with a longer side of no more than 20 cm, and no more than twice the shorter side.[9]

H.
Monitor Factors and Field Size Dependence Factors

After all of the above parameters have been specified, the data tables should include a list of square field sizes versus either monitor factors, dose rates, or field size dependence factors.

An integrating dosimeter built into a treatment unit measures accumulating dose in terms of digital units which "click" off on either a mechanical or electrical counter. These digital units are called **monitor units**, which we shall refer to as μ (the Greek letter mu, for monitor unit).

By adjusting the dosimeter circuitry, it is possible to make one monitor unit correspond to one cGy delivered at some specified distance for a specified field size. The specified distance is normally the source to isocenter distance (or in some cases this distance + d_{max}), and the specified field size is normally 10 x 10 cm.

If the monitor is adjusted for this one specific pair of variables, then if either the distance or field size are changed, one monitor unit will correspond to either more or less than one cGy, since the monitor is unaware of the field size or treatment distance being used.

For example, if the monitor on the Clinac-4 is adjusted to click once for each cGy for a 10 x 10 cm field at 80 cm SAD, it will click once every 0.965 cGy for a 6 x 6 cm field at the same distance. If we divide the number of cGy delivered by the number of monitor units counted for any exposure under these conditions, we get:

$$\frac{0.965 \; cGy}{1 \; monitor \; unit}$$

This quantity (0.965) is an example of a monitor factor. **The monitor factor is defined as the absorbed dose per monitor unit at d_{max} in a maxiphantom.** Each field size has its own monitor factor. The monitor factor will also be different at distances other than the calibration distance, and can be approximated by using the inverse square law. The scheme for finding the monitor factor for a field A x B at distance Z is:

$$monitor \; factor \; for \; field \; A \cdot B \; at \; calibration \; distance \left(\frac{calibration \; distance}{Z}\right)^2$$

For example, on the Clinac-4, where the calibration distance is 80 cm, and the monitor factor for a 6 x 6 cm field is 0.965, then the monitor factor for a 6 x 6 cm field at 85 cm would be:

$$0.965 \left(\frac{80}{85}\right)^2 = 0.855$$

A field size factor is the dose per monitor unit (or the dose per minute) for a field A x B divided by the dose per monitor unit (or the dose per minute) for a 10 x 10 cm field at the calibration distance.

While you may use a monitor factor directly in dose planning, in order to use a field size factor you must first multiply it by the dose rate for a 10 x 10 cm field. Observe:

$$(\textit{Field size factor}) \cdot (\textit{dose for } 10 \times 10 \; \textit{cm field})$$

$$= \left(\frac{\textit{dose rate for field } A \cdot B}{\textit{dose rate for } 10 \times 10 \; \textit{field}} \right) \cdot (\textit{dose rate for } 10 \times 10 \; \textit{cm field})$$

$$= \textit{dose rate for field } A \cdot B$$

Thus an alternative to listing field size factors is to simply list the dose rates of each field involved. The same number of figures is involved.

References

1. Attix, F.H. *Introduction to Radiological Physics and Radiation Dosimetry*, John Wiley & Sons, New York, 1986, pp. 358-360.
2. Massey, J.B. *Manual of Dosimetry in Radiotherapy*, Technical Report Series #110, International Atomic Energy Agency, Vienna, 1970, pp. 12-13.
3. Johns, H.E. & Cunningham, J.R. *The Physics of Radiology*, 4th Edition, Charles C. Thomas, Springfield, 1983, pp. 235-240.
4. Khan, F.M. *The Physics of Radiation Therapy*, Williams & Wilkins, Baltimore, 1984, Chapter 6.
5. Selman, J. *The Basic Physics of Radiation Therapy*, 2nd Edition, Charles C. Thomas, Springfield, 1976, pp. 177-188.
6. AAPM Task Group 21. "A Protocol for the Determination of Absorbed Dose for High-Energy Photon and Electron Beams," *Med Phys* 10 (6), pp. 741-771.
7. *X-Rays and Gamma Rays with Maximum Photon Energies Between 0.6 and 50 MV*, Report 14, International Commission on Radiation Units and Measurements, Washington, D.C., United States National Bureau of Standards, 1969, Appendix B.
8. *Central Axis Depth Dose Data for Use in Radiotherapy*, British Journal of Radiology Supplement 17, 1983, Table AA.2, pp. 112-113.
9. Ibid., Appendix A, pp. 105-114.
10. Ibid., p. 146.

Dosimetry of Source-Skin Distance (SSD) Techniques

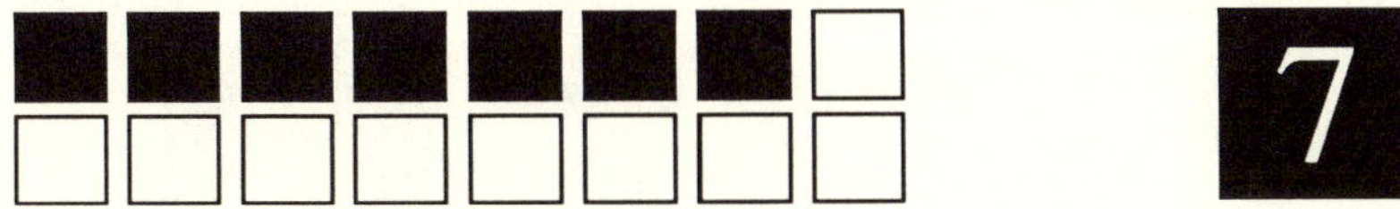

7

A. Output Data for SSD Techniques
B. Peak Scatter Factor (PSF), Backscatter Factor (BF)
C. Depth Dose Fraction (Percent Depth Dose)
D. Factors Governing Depth Dose Fraction
E. Variation in Depth Dose Fraction with SSD
F. Calculating a Treatment Duration to Deliver a Prescription Dose to a Specified Point on the Central Ray in a Single Field
G. Calculation of Dose to Points Other Than the Prescription Point
H. Using Non-Standard SSD
I. Calculation of Dose with Opposing Equally Weighted Fields

Source to Skin Distance (SSD) techniques are treatment techniques in which the normalization point is at the depth of maximum dose (d_{max}) and the patient set-up techniques (field size, location, and alignment) are referenced to the patient's skin. **Simple dosimetry** refers to treatment planning based on central ray data; i.e., one dimensional data. No isodose summation is performed.

A.
Output Data for SSD Techniques

Machine data tables listing dose rates or monitor factors at a given SSD are preferred. This means that the normalization point is further from the source than the reference distance, SSD, by a distance equal to d_{max}.

For example, if you wish to treat at 80 cm SSD, the most convenient data table would be one listed as 80 cm SSD, with the normalization point at 81 cm for 4 MV or 80.5 cm for cobalt-60. If this is not the case, you should make the appropriate inverse square law correction as discussed in Chapter 6, Section H.

Data tables listing dose rates in a miniphantom may also be used if you are careful to include the peak scatter factor or back-scatter factor (described below) in the calculations.

B.
Peak Scatter Factor (PSF), Backscatter Factor (BF)

$$PSF = \frac{dose\ at\ d_{max}\ in\ maxiphantom}{dose\ in\ miniphantom*}$$

For x-rays with peak voltages no more than 400 kV, the peak scatter factor is called the backscatter factor (BF).[1]

Peak scatter factors are always greater than one. This is because the numerator of the above definition involves all of the radiation involved in the denominator, plus radiation scattered back to the point of reference. Thus the numerator will always be greater than the denominator, and the PSF will be greater than unity. For example, if the PSF = 1.06, this implies that 0.06 (or 6%), of the radiation reaching the reference point is backscatter.

Backscatter is not the same thing as the backscatter factor.[2,3] Backscatter is any radiation which has scattered through an angle greater than 90 degrees. All the scatter may not reach the reference point, either because it is headed in the wrong direction, or because it is absorbed before it gets there.

Peak scatter and backscatter factors are independent of SSD. Scatter mainly depends on the beam quality and field size.

In order to contribute to the PSF or BF, the radiation must (a) backscatter, and (b) return to the reference point. The probability of (a) or (b) does not depend in any way on how far the photon had to travel from the source.

The factors which determine the magnitude of PSF or BF are: nature of the radiation, field size and shape (equivalent square), nature of the absorber (usually muscle tissue unless otherwise specified), and thickness of the absorber (considered to be "semi-infinite" unless otherwise specified).

In general, the larger the equivalent square, the greater the PSF or BF, although the relationship is not linear (i.e. not in direct proportion).[4]

The denser the medium, the smaller the PSF or BF, although you do not generally consider media other than water, muscle or fat, since the buildup point rarely lies in other media.

The thicker the absorber, the higher the PSF or BF, up to the point at which the medium becomes a maxiphantom (or

---

* for same exposure, field size, and distance from source.

semi-infinite). After that point thickness is no longer a determining factor, by definition (see Chapter 6, section A).

The relationship between BF and radiation type is more complex (see Figure 7.1).

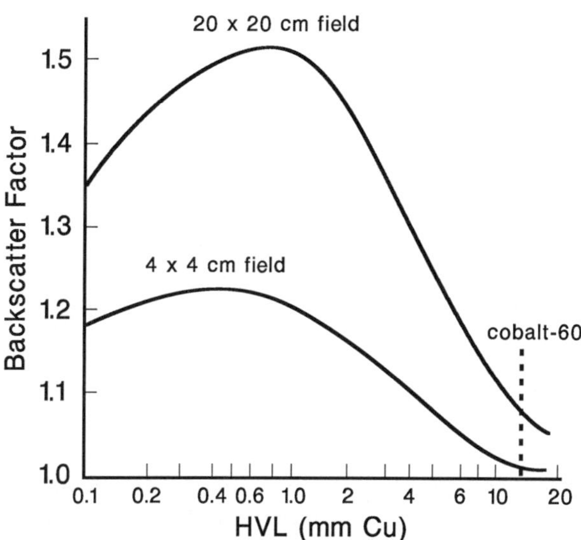

Figure 7.1. Backscatter factors at various energies for two field sizes.

Observe that as you proceed from a lower to a higher energy (as indicated by an increasing half-value layer), the backscatter factor for a given field size increases to a maximum value at a HVL between 0.5 mm and 1 mm of copper (Cu), whereupon it begins falling again. It will never quite reach 1.0.

Two factors cause this maximum. First, the likelihood of backscatter is always less at higher photon energies. Backscatter alone would cause a decrease in the PSF or BF at higher and higher energies. Second, for softer radiations, the scattered photons are more apt to be absorbed before reaching the point of maximum dose. That is, the percent reaching that point increases for harder radiations. Thus we have both an increasing function and a decreasing function at work, which gives us a maximum in the BF curve. The peak just happens to occur in the low orthovoltage (intermediate voltage) therapy range.

For different field sizes, the shape of the graph is similar, but the values of BF are larger or smaller.[5] Note that the BF is nearly 1.5 for low orthovoltage and medium to large fields; i.e., the error involved in ignoring this factor can be extremely serious.

C.
Depth Dose Fraction (Percent Depth Dose)

The depth dose fraction (ddf) is defined as follows:

$$ddf = \frac{\text{dose at depth of interest}}{\text{dose at } d_{max}}, \text{ in the same field}$$

The dose at the depth of interest may be on the central ray or elsewhere. The point of interest may be deeper than d_{max}, or it may lie between the surface and d_{max}. It may, in fact, be the normalization point, in which case ddf is equal to 1. The normalization point itself will be on the central ray.

Depth dose fractions are always less than or equal to one.

To see how you use the ddf, simply rewrite the defining equation as follows:

$$\text{Dose at } d_{max} = \frac{\text{dose at depth of interest}}{ddf}$$

since you will normally know both the ddf (from the tables) and the dose at some depth of interest (from the dose prescription) and will want to determine the dose at d_{max} in order to determine treatment duration (in either time or monitor units).

Percent depth dose is simply ddf x 100%. It is really rather pointless to use percent depth dose, since the quantity always enters into the calculations in the form of a fraction.

D.
Factors Governing Depth Dose Fraction

The magnitude of ddf is determined by radiation type, the specific treatment unit involved, field size and shape, depth, and SSD.

Higher energy radiation will involve higher ddfs, because of its greater penetration. If all other factors are equal, a 4 MV beam will have a larger ddf than a cobalt-60 beam.

It is also true, however, that no two treatment units are alike, and the depth dose fractions for two different cobalt units may be slightly different. This is certainly true for linacs. Ideally, if the time and personnel are available, a set of depth dose fractions should be measured for each individual machine. Failing this, "standard" depth dose tables, which are found, for example, in Johns & Cunningham or in BJR Supplement #17 may be used, resulting in errors of usually only a few percent.[6,7]

Depth dose fractions will vary with field size and shape (i.e. equivalent squares) because of the increase in scattered radiation with larger fields. Since scattered radiation is more important at depths of clinical interest than at the d_{max}, ddfs will increase with increasing field size.[8]

Obviously, ddf is a function of depth.[9] Actually, ddf **increases** with depth from the surface to d_{max}, then continuously decreases.

E.
Variation in Depth Dose Fraction with SSD

While it is true that the dose rate should **decrease** at greater SSD according to the inverse square law, the depth dose fraction actually **increases** with greater SSD. To understand why, consider that the ddf is less than one (except at the normalization point, where it is equal to one) because of two effects.

The first effect is **tissue attenuation**, which is the removal of radiation by interaction with the tissue between the d_{max} and the depth of interest. The second is the **inverse square law factor** since the point at d_{max} and the depth of interest are at different distances from the source.

The first of these factors, tissue attenuation, is the same at any SSD, since a given thickness of tissue will remove the same fraction of incident radiation regardless of its distance from the source. Thus the variation in ddf is due solely to the inverse square law factor. If we limit ourselves to depths beyond that of d_{max}, it is easily seen that the inverse square law factor is always less than one:

$$inverse\ square\ factor\ (ISF) = \left(\frac{SSD + d_{max}}{SSD + depth}\right)^2$$

Thus, the closer to one we make the value of ISF, the greater the ddf. The maximum value of ddf is limited to the tissue attenuation factor.

The inverse square law factor will be close to one if the numerator and denominator are about the same size. This will occur if the SSD is much larger than the depth. Consider that if SSD is 10 cm, d_{max} is 1 cm, and the depth is 10 cm, the inverse square law factor is much less than one:

$$ISF = \left(\frac{10 + 1}{10 + 10}\right)^2 = \left(\frac{11}{20}\right)^2 = 0.30$$

whereas with the same depth of 10 cm and d_{max} of 1 cm, but an SSD of 100 cm:

$$ISF = \left(\frac{100 + 1}{100 + 10}\right)^2 = \left(\frac{101}{110}\right)^2 = 0.84$$

If the SSD were one mile, consider the unimportant difference between numerator and denominator - one mile versus one mile plus 4 inches.

Since the inverse square law factor increases at greater SSD, and the tissue attenuation factor does not change, the ddf must increase.

A method of calculating a new ddf at a given depth for a new SSD using the known ddf at the same depth is derived as follows:

$$ddf = \text{inverse square factor (ISF)} \cdot \text{tissue attenuation factor (TAF)}$$

$$ddf_o = (ISF)_o \cdot TAF$$

$$ddf_n = (ISF)_n \cdot TAF$$

(where subscripts "o" and "n" represent "old" and "new"). The second expression can be written:

$$ddf_n = (ISF)_n \cdot TAF \cdot \frac{(ISF)_o}{(ISF)_o} = \frac{(ISF)_n}{(ISF)_o} \cdot (TAF \cdot ISF_o)$$

$$= \frac{(ISF)_n}{(ISF)_o} \cdot ddf_o = ddf_o \cdot \frac{\left(\dfrac{SSD_n + d_{max}}{SSD_n + depth}\right)^2}{\left(\dfrac{SSD_o + d_{max}}{SSD_o + depth}\right)^2}$$

so:

$$ddf_n = ddf_o \left(\frac{SSD_n + d_{max}}{SSD_n + depth}\right)^2 \cdot \left(\frac{SSD_o + depth}{SSD_o + d_{max}}\right)^2$$

The quantity on the right is called **Mayneord F-factor**.[10]

The use of the inverse square law in the Mayneord F-factor assumes that all radiation contributing to ddf is coming from the source, which is of course not true, since scattered radiation originates in the patient and at the collimator. Thus the F-factor contains a built-in error which is greater when scattered radiation is more important. This is true for large field sizes and/or low energy. Therefore the F-factor is most applicable for small and medium fields, and high energy photons. It gives reasonably good results for cobalt-60 units and linacs. For large differences in SSD, a further correction for the effect of field may be desired (see Appendix B of Reference 1).

F.

Calculating a Treatment Duration to Deliver a Prescription Dose to a Specified Point on The Central Ray in a Single Field

Treatment duration may be either a time in minutes and seconds (if the exposure is terminated by a timer), or it may be a number of monitor units (μ) if the exposure is terminated by an integrating dosimeter, as on a linear accelerator.

A **prescription dose** is the dose decided upon in advance by the radiation therapist to be delivered to a point of primary interest.

We will use the following symbols in the interest of brevity:

CAL   the number from machine data tables, representing a calibration, for the specified treatment unit, SSD, and field size. It may be a monitor factor, a number of cGy per minute in air or in a maxiphantom at d_{max}, or a number of roentgens per minute in air, depending on the type of calibration.

ddf   depth dose fraction

PSF   peak scatter factor for the specified field size

BF   backscatter factor for the the specified field size

f   the roentgen to Gy conversion factor

$\mathbf{D_p}$ prescription dose (Gy or cGy)

T   treatment duration in minutes or number of monitor units.

In the following examples, the appropriate data will be taken from the tables in the appendices.

Example 7.1:

Using data tables in Appendix B, calculate the time required to deliver 3 Gy to a depth of 5 mm from a superficial x-ray unit with a half-value layer (HVL) of 1 mm Al through a field size of 4 x 8 cm at the skin. The SSD is 20 cm.

From the data tables, Appendix B, CAL equals 120 cGy/min, and d_{max} is on the surface. The depth dose chart for HVL is 1 mm Al, 20 cm SSD (or TSD, target to skin distance) is found in Appendix B. Also on this sheet are the f-factor for muscle and the backscatter factors. For a 4 x 8 cm field the equivalent square is 2(4 x 8)/(4 + 8) = 64/12 = 5.3 cm (the accurate number is 5.4, which is taken from Reference 1, p. 112). (For now, equate equivalent square with equivalent circle.) Interpolating ddf between 4.4 cm and 5.6 cm in the table, the interpolated value of ddf is:

$$\frac{5.3 - 4.4}{5.6 - 4.4} = 0.75$$

so the desired $ddf_{5.3}$:

$$= ddf_{4.4} + 0.75\,(ddf_{5.6} - ddf_{4.4})$$
$$= 0.792 + 0.75\,(0.798 - 0.792)$$
$$= 0.892 + 0.75\,(0.006)$$
$$= 0.792 + 0.005$$
$$= 0.797$$

Similarly, the interpolated backscatter factor for the equivalent circle of 5.3 cm is:

$$BF_{5.3} = BF_{4.4} + 0.75\,(BF_{5.6} - BF_{4.4})$$
$$= 1.13 + 0.75\,(1.15 - 1.13)$$
$$= 1.15$$

Knowing the ddf and prescribed dose (D_p), you can calculate the dose at d_{max} as follows: f = 0.903 rads/R
Dose at d_{max} (skin):

$$= D_p\,/ddf\;(from\ definition\ of\ ddf)$$
$$= 3.0\ Gy/0.797$$
$$= 3.76\ Gy$$

Since f = 0.903 rads/ R = 0.903 cGy/R, the dose rate at skin:

$$= (exposure\ rate\ in\ air) \cdot (BF) \cdot (f)$$
$$= (120R/min)\ x\ (1.15)\ x\ (0.903)\ cGy/R$$
$$= 1.25\ Gy/min$$

So the required time is T:

$$= 3.76\ Gy/\ 1.25\ Gy/min$$
$$= 3.01\ min$$

Note that the calculation procedure is:

$$T = \frac{D_p}{(cal) \cdot (BF) \cdot (ddf)}$$

Example 7.2:

Using the data tables in Appendix C, calculate the time needed to deliver 2 Gy to a depth of 5 cm through a 10 x 15 cm field, using a cobalt-60 unit. Assume the date to be 9/15/78, and that the SSD is 80 cm.

The only differences between this and Example 7.1 are:

(a) CAL is given in cGy/min in a maxiphantom, so no BF or f is required.

(b) CAL is a function of time, since the cobalt source decays. Thus:

$$T = \frac{d_p}{(CAL) \cdot (ddf)}$$

The equivalent square is:

$$\frac{2(10 \text{ x } 15)}{(10 + 15)} = 12 \; cm$$

From the data tables, the field size factor for a 12 x 12 cm field is 1.015, and the 10 x 10 cm dose rate on 9/15/78 was 68.4 cGy/min. So CAL = 1.015 x 68.4 cGy/min = 69.4 cGy/min.

From the depth dose table for this cobalt unit in Appendix C, ddf (12 x 12 cm, 5 cm) = 0.805. Thus:

$$T = \frac{2 \; Gy}{69.4 \; cGy/min \text{ x } 0.805} = 3.58 \; min.$$

But, note that there is a timer correction of 0.03 minute for this unit, to be subtracted from the calculated time. Thus:

$$T = 3.58 \; min \; - 0.03 \; min \; = 3.55 \; min.$$

Example 7.3:

Calculate the monitor setting required to deliver 250 cGy to a depth of 10 cm through a 10 x 10 cm field at 79 cm target to skin distance (TSD, which has the same meaning as SSD) using the Clinac-4. Obtain CAL directly from the depth dose table, Appendix D.

You do not have to calculate an equivalent square for a square field. From the depth dose sheet, the monitor factor CAL = 1.00 cGy/μ and ddf is 0.601 for a depth of 10 cm.

$$T = \frac{Dp}{(CAL) \cdot (ddf)} = \frac{2.5 \; Gy}{(1 \; cGy /\mu) \text{ x} (0.601)} = 416 \; \mu$$

G.
Calculation of Dose to Points Other than the Prescription Point

Having calculated the treatment duration for a predetermined dose to a single point, it is often required to find what dose is being delivered to other points in the same irradiated field. If the ddf's at these other points are known, this may be done using the simple proportion:

$$\frac{D_x}{D_p} = \frac{ddf_x}{ddf_p} \quad or \quad D_x = \frac{ddf_x}{D_p \cdot ddf_p}$$

Most often, the dose at d_{max} (often called the "given dose") is immediately sought. The reason is that this dose is usually to normal tissue, and acts as a limiting factor in the case of a single field. $D_x = D_{max}$, $ddf_x = 1.0$. So:

$$D_{max} = D_p\left(\frac{1}{ddf_p}\right), \quad or \quad D_p = (D_{max}) \cdot (ddf)$$

Example 7.4:

For the case in Example 7.3, find the dose given at d_{max} and to a depth of 14 cm on the central axis.

The treatment duration has already been found. It was decided to deliver 2.5 Gy to a depth of 10 cm, TSD = 79 cm, field size = 10 x 10 cm. The ddf for 10 cm was 0.601.

$$D_{max} = \frac{D_p}{ddf_p} = \frac{2.5\,Gy}{0.601} = 4.16\,Gy$$

The depth dose chart indicates that ddf equals 0.465 at 14 cm depth.

$$D_{14cm} = D_p\left(\frac{ddf_{14}}{ddf_p}\right) = 2.5\,Gy\left(\frac{0.465}{0.601}\right) = 1.93\,Gy$$

H.
Using Non-Standard SSD

On occasion you must plan a patient treatment using an SSD other than that for which the ddf table is valid. In such a case, you should make the following two corrections:
(a) correct CAL by means of the inverse square law.
(b) correct ddf using the Mayneord F-factor, if no depth dose

data are available at the new SSD. As an alternative, you may interpolate if the new SSD is not different from the old SSD by more than 10 cm and lies between two SSD's for which ddf's are available. This is an approximation, since interpolation is only valid for linear relationships, and the variation of ddf with SSD is non-linear.

Correction of CAL is a two step process. First you must decide which of the field sizes on the calibration sheet corresponds to the field size in question at the new SSD. See Figure 7.2.

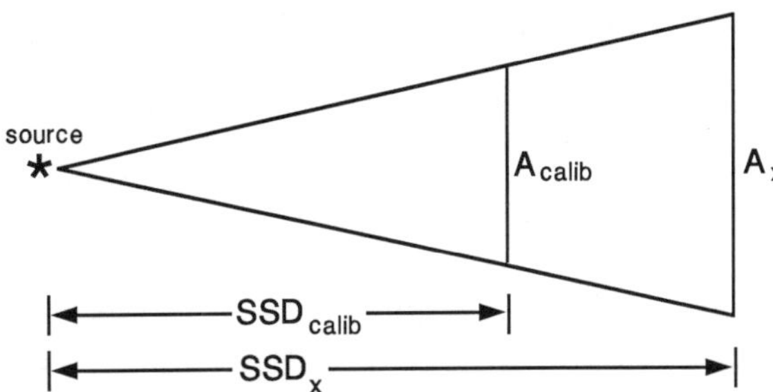

A_{calib} and A_x are the equivalent square sides at the calibration SSD and the new SSD respectively. A_x and SSD_x are known for the specific case in question, and SSD_{calib} is indicated in the data tables. According to proportions using similar triangles:

$$A_{calib} = A_x \left(\frac{SSD_{calib}}{SSD_x} \right)$$

This is again an approximation, since calibration numbers for different field sizes vary because of scattering both at the collimator and within the patient. While the effect of scattering from the collimator onto the patient is affected by the SSD, scattering within the patient is not. The most accurate answer lies somewhere between the result of the above procedure and no size correction at all.

Having decided on a field size to read from the calibration sheet, you must now correct CAL to the new SSD, by means of the inverse square law:

$$CAL_n = CAL_o \left(\frac{SSD_o + d_{max}}{SSD_n + d_{max}} \right)^2$$

Example 7.5:

Using the cobalt output data in Appendix C, find CAL_n for a 10 x 15 cm field at an SSD of 90 cm (date 1/15/79).

The equivalent square is:

$$\frac{2(10 \times 15)}{(10 + 15)} = \frac{300}{25} = 12\ cm$$

$$A_{calib} = A_x\left(\frac{SSD_{calib}}{SSD_x}\right) = 12\left(\frac{80}{90}\right) = 10.67\ cm$$

which means we must find CAL_o for a 10.67 cm equivalent square on the output table. Interpolation gives a field size factor of 1.006, and at 1/15/79 the dose rate for a 10 x 10 cm field is 65.5 cGy/min. Thus: CAL_o = 1.006 x 65.5 cGy/min = 65.9 cGy/min. Applying the inverse square law:

$$CAL_n = CAL_o\left(\frac{SSD_o + d_{max}}{SSD_n + d_{max}}\right)^2 = 65.9\ cGy/min\left(\frac{80 + 0.5}{90 + 0.5}\right)^2 = 52.1\ cGy/min$$

Example 7.6:

> For the above, find the result if the first step is omitted; i.e., if you begin with a 12 x 12 field from the output tables.

Field size factor for a 12 x12 cm field = 1.015, dose rate for a 10 x 10 cm field is 65.5 cGy/min. CAL_o = 1.015 x 65.5 cGy/min = 65.5 cGy/min,

$$CAL_n = 65.5\ cGy/min\left(\frac{80.5}{90.5}\right)^2 = 52.6\ cGy/min$$

which differs from the previous answer by only 1.0%.

Example 7.7:

> Find the monitor setting for the Clinac-4 which will deliver 2 Gy to a depth of 6 cm through a 10 x 15 cm field at an SSD of 90 cm.

The equivalent square was found in the last example to be 12. The corresponding field size at 79 cm is:

$$A_{calib} = 12\left(\frac{79}{90}\right) = 10.5\ cm$$

The monitor factor (CAL) from the depth dose table, Appendix D, for a 10.5 cm effective square is 1.003 cGy/μ. Applying the inverse square correction:

$$CAL_{90} = 1.003\left(\frac{79 + 1}{90 + 1}\right)^2 = 0.775\ cGy\ /\mu$$

The depth dose fraction at 79 cm SSD for a 12 x 12 cm field, at the depth of 6 cm is 0.778 (from the depth dose chart, Appendix D).

Applying the Mayncord F-factor:

$$ddf_{90} = 0.778 \left(\frac{90 + 1}{90 + 6}\right)^2 \cdot \left(\frac{79 + 6}{79 + 1}\right)^2 = 0.789$$

Thus:

$$T = \frac{D_p}{(CAL) \cdot (ddf)} = \frac{2\,Gy}{(0.775\,cGy\,/\,\mu) \cdot (0.789)} = 327\,\mu$$

I.
Calculation of Dose With Opposing Equally Weighted Fields

Opposing fields are those whose central rays coincide but which enter on opposite sides of the patient.

Equal weight means, for SSD calculations, that each of the two fields delivers the same dose to its own d_{max}. The fields are usually, but not always, the same size.

The calculation procedure is exactly as already described for single fields, since each field of the opposing pair is indeed a single field. It must be remembered, however, that each point in the tissue is receiving dose from both fields.

The advantage of opposing ports with equal weight is that the entire volume between buildup points receives an almost homogeneous dose. This is best seen in Example 7.8.

Example 7.8:

Two opposing equally weighted ports are used to treat a patient section 16 cm thick. The fields are 15 x 15 cm fields at 79 cm SSD from a Clinac-4. Both fields are treated each day, and a combined dose of 2 Gy is desired at midline.

Since the prescription point is halfway through the patient and the fields are the same size, each field will deliver 1 Gy to the prescription point if equal doses are given to the buildup points. You might first calculate the treatment duration to accomplish this. This will be left as an exercise, since what we desire in this example is a comparison of doses at various depths, in order to see the degree of homogeneity.

We will calculate the dose to points A, B, C, D, and E in Figure 7.3. For this we will need the following data from Appendix D:

$$ddf_1 \text{ at } 1 \text{ cm} = 1.00$$
$$ddf_4 \text{ at } 4 \text{ cm} = 0.873$$
$$ddf_8 \text{ at } 8 \text{ cm} = 0.074$$
$$ddf_{12} \text{ at } 12 \text{ cm} = 0.559$$
$$ddf15 \text{ at } 15 \text{ cm} = 0.467$$

By summing the dose from both fields (found in the table below) to each point, you find: dose to A and E, 2.08 Gy; dose to B and D, 2.03 Gy; dose to C, 2.00 Gy.

Thus the deviation from homogeneity is only 4% along the entire central ray from d_{max} on one side to d_{max} on the other side.

Figure 7.3.
Parallel opposed
fields.

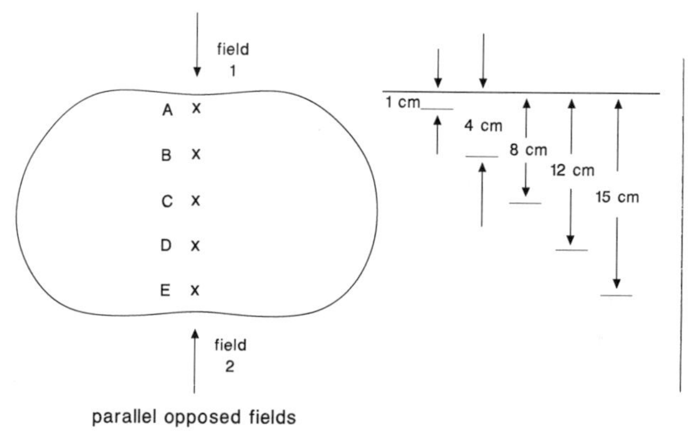

Field 1

	Depth (cm)	ddf	Dose* (cGy)
Point A	1	1.00	142
Point B	4	0.873	124
Point C	8	0.704	100
Point D	12	0.559	79
Point E	15	0.467	66

Field 2

	Depth (cm)	ddf	Dose* (cGy)
Point A	15	0.467	66
Point B	12	0.559	79
Point C	8	0.704	100
Point D	4	0.873	124
Point E	1	1.00	142

* Dose is calculated from $D_x = D_p \left(\dfrac{ddf_x}{ddf_p} \right)$

This homogeneity will be good for large fields, high energy radiation and thin body sections. It is not as good for small fields, softer radiations, and thick body parts. To see this we will do another example.

Example 7.9:

Do the same procedure as above, except with 5 x 5 cm cobalt fields at 80 cm SSD, through a 30 cm thick patient.

We will do points at 0.5, 7, and 15 cm from each side. For this we will need (from Appendix C):

$$ddf_{0.5} = 1.00$$
$$ddf_7 = 0.646$$
$$ddf_{15} = 0.343$$
$$ddf_{22} = 0.196$$
$$ddf_{29.5} = 0.112$$

Here the maximum departure from homogeneity is 63%, which is obviously not good.

Field 1

	Depth (cm)	ddf	Dose* (cGy)
Point A	0.5	1.00	292
Point B	7	0.646	188
Point C	15	0.343	100
Point D	22	0.196	57
Point E	29.5	0.122	33

Field 2

	Depth (cm)	ddf	Dose* (cGy)
Point A	29.5	0.112	33
Point B	22	0.196	57
Point C	15	0.343	100
Point D	7	0.646	188
Point E	0.5	1.00	292

References

1. *Central Axis Depth Dose Data for Use in Radiotherapy*, British Journal of Radiology Supplement 17, 1983, p. 143.
2. Ibid., p. 146.
3. Johns, H.E. & Cunningham, J.R. *The Physics of Radiology*, 4th Edition, Charles C. Thomas, Springfield, 1983, pp. 338, 347.
4. *Measurement of Absorbed Dose in a Phantom Irradiated by a Single Beam of X or Gamma Rays*, Report 23, International Commission on Radiation Units and Measurements, Washington, D.C., 1973, pp. 11-13.
5. Johns & Cunningham, p. 348.
6. *Central Axis Depth Dose Data for Use in Radiotherapy*, British Journal of Radiology Supplement 11, Appendix D, 1972, p. 113. See also BJR Supplement #17, page 130.
7. Johns & Cunningham, Appendix B.
8. Ibid., p. 351.
9. Ibid., p. 349.
10. Mayneord, W. & Lamerton, L. "A Survey of Depth Dose Data," *British Journal of Radiology*, 14:255, 1941.

Dosimetry of Simple Isocentric (SAD) Techniques

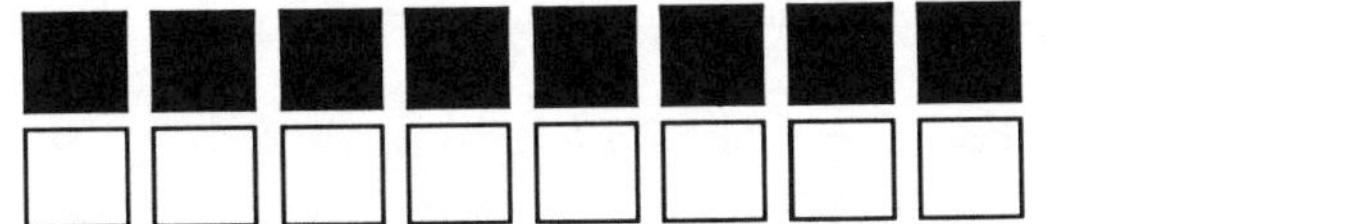

Source to Axis Distance (SAD) techniques can be used with radiation units where the source can be positioned at various angles around the patient. The axis around which the source rotates is called the isocentric axis. The gantry is the mechanism that supports the radiation source. SAD techniques may be used, however, whether the normalization point is on the axis (isocenter) or not.

With SAD techniques, the normalization point is usually (though not always) located within the target (tumor) volume, rather than at depth of maximum dose (d_{max}). The field size is always specified at the axis. For SAD techniques, the field size on the skin can be found using the proportion for similar triangles which we used in Chapter 6, Section H.

The field size on the skin is only of secondary importance. It serves as a check on the accuracy of the patient set-up procedure in the treatment room.

Depth dose fractions and peak scatter (backscatter) factors are not used with SAD techniques, since these are referenced at the buildup point. One of the following three ratios are used in place of the depth dose fraction: TAR (tissue to air ratio), TMR (tissue to maximium ratio) or TPR (tissue to phantom ratio).

A.
Tissue-Air Ratio (TAR)

TAR is defined as follows:[1] for a given treatment unit and energy, at a specified depth and a specified field size:

$$TAR = \frac{dose\ at\ specified\ depth\ in\ tissue}{dose\ at\ same\ SAD\ miniphantom\ placed\ in\ air}$$

TAR is also equal to ratio dose rates measured under the same conditions. See Figure 8.1 for the detailed setup of TAR.

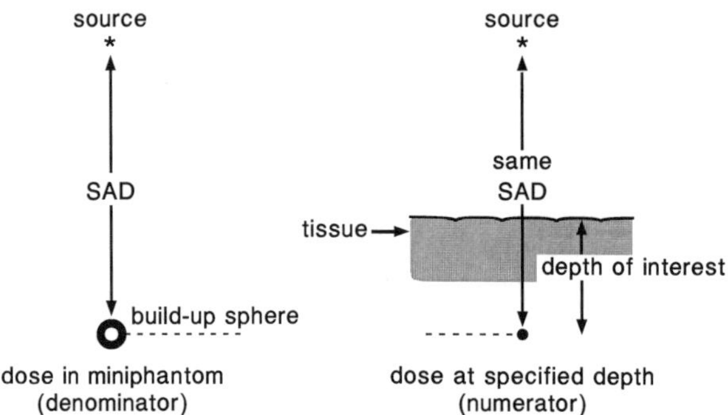

Notice that the above definition is a maxiphantom dose divided by a miniphantom dose. This being the case, the scatter has an effect on the magnitude of the numerator, but not the denominator, of the fraction. Thus the peak scatter factor (PSF) or backscatter factor (BF) is inherently contained in the TAR, and need not be introduced separately into the calculations. In fact, if the depth of reference in the numerator is the depth of maximum dose (which is possible, but rarely clinically practical), then the TAR is numerically equal to the peak scatter factor (or backscatter factor). This same characteristic of the TAR makes its use troublesome when using a monitor factor, (i.e., when using a treatment unit with an integrating dose monitor), since the monitor factor contains information due to scatter from both the tissue and the collimator. If TAR's are used in the same calculations with monitor factors, then the tissue peak scatter factor (or backscatter factor) would enter twice into the calculations, both times in disguise. This would, of course, result in an error.

B.
Tissue-Maximium Ratio (TMR)

TMR is defined for a specific treatment unit and energy, and for a specified depth and a specified field size as follows:[2,3]

$$TMR = \frac{dose\ at\ specified\ depth\ in\ tissue}{dose\ at\ same\ SAD\ at\ d_{max}\ in\ maxiphantom}$$

See Figure 8.2 for detailed set-up of TMR measurement.

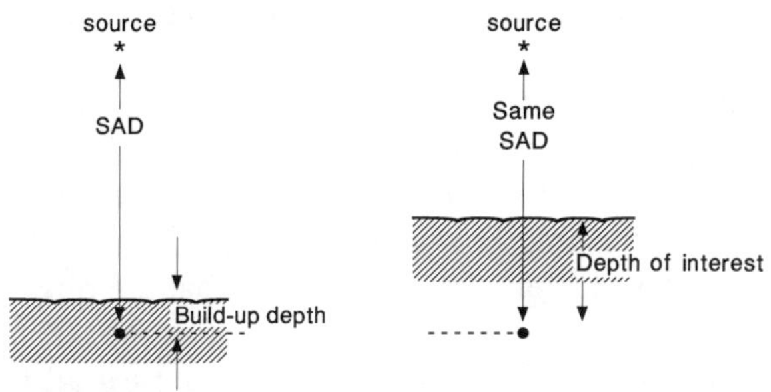

Figure 8.2. Set-up for tissue-maximum ratio measurement.

The difference between TAR and TMR is in the denominator. In TMR, both numerator and denominator are maxiphantom doses, and thus both contain the same information about tissue scatter. Therefore, the two peak scatter factors will cancel out in the TMR. The TMR is specifically designed to be used with a monitor factor, however, and monitor factors implicitly contain the backscatter, so again one need not introduce PSF explicitly into the calculations.

The value of TMR at d_{max} is 1.00. This can readily be seen from the definition above.

C.
Tissue-Phantom Ratio (TPR)

TPR is defined for a given treatment unit and energy at a specified depth and a specified field size as follows:[4]

$$TPR = \frac{dose\ at\ specified\ depth\ in\ tissue}{dose\ at\ reference\ depth\ in\ maxiphantom,\ at\ same\ SAD}$$

See Figure 8.3 for detailed setup for TPR measurement.

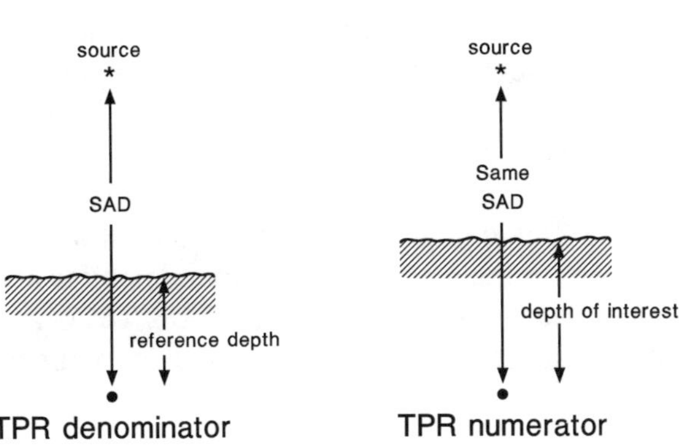

Figure 8.3. Set-up for tissue-phantom ratio measurement.

Again, the differences among TAR, TMR, and TPR are all in the denominator. While the reference point in the maxiphantom must be at buildup for TMR, it may be at any specified point for TPR. Thus TMR is a special subclass of TPR. TPR is seldom used clinically, except in the following sense, best shown by example.

The depth of d_{max} for 10 MV photons from the Clinac-18 is nominally 2.0 cm, but in fact varies from about 2.5 cm for small fields down to about 1.5 cm for large fields. If we were to specify TMR's for this unit, we would have to use a different reference depth for each field size (remember that the reference depth for TMR is at d_{max}). This would be cumbersome. The reference depth which appears on TMR tables is 2.5 cm for all field sizes. Since this is not necessarily at d_{max}, what we are calling a TMR is really a TPR with a reference point close to d_{max}.

D.
Comments on TAR, TMR, and TPR

(1) The value of the TMR is never greater than one.

(2) The value of the TAR can have a greater value than one close to d_{max}, but is never greater than the peak scatter factor (or backscatter factor) for the field size used.

(3) The value of a TPR has no upper limit. The deeper the reference depth, the greater the TPR.

(4) Output tables for use with TAR's must involve measurements made with a miniphantom at a specified distance from the source.

(5) A calibration sheet for use with TMR's uses measurements made in a maxiphantom, either with the reference chamber located at d_{max}, or preferably with the chamber at the depth recommended by AAPM calibration protocol and ICRU 14, in which case the output at d_{max} is determined by calculation (see Chapter 6, Section F).[5,6]

(6) A calibration sheet for use with TPR's uses measurements made in a maxiphantom with the reference chamber either at the reference depth specified in the TPR denominator, or calculated for this depth after measurement at the specific AAPM protocol depth.

(7) Note especially that the TAR, TPR, and TMR do not involve the inverse square law. The inverse square law involves two distances, from the source to two separate points at different distances. The above definitions of TAR, TMR, and TPR specifically state that the numerator and denominator involve

the same point (i.e., the same SAD) under two different conditions of absorption. Thus the inverse square law factor is always 1.0. For this reason:

(8) TAR, TMR and TPR are independent of distance from the source. For a given treatment unit and energy, the same tables can be used at any SAD.

E.
Tables for TAR, TMR, and TPR

Examples of each kind of table are located in Appendix B, although the TMR table for the 10 MV photon of the Clinac-18 is really a TPR table, as explained above.

The parameters for the tables are much the same as for a depth dose table, with the exception that no treatment distance is specified, since these variables are independent of treatment distance. (Of course, the treatment distance is still important in determining the monitor factor to be used with the selected TAR, TMR, or TPR.)

Compare values of TMR and depth dose fraction for the 4 MV machine. Note that both have a value of 1.0 at 1 cm, d_{max}, but the TMR at other depths is significantly larger than the ddf. This is because greater depths in the ddf table represent points further and further from the source. If you decide to use the TMR table with monitor factors for an 80 cm SAD, however, then every value in the TMR table corresponds to a point 80 cm from the source. If you used a monitor factor suitable for 100 cm SAD, then every TMR would correspond to a distance of 100 cm, etc.

F.
Calculating Timer or Monitor Setting to Deliver a Prescription Dose to the Isocenter with a Single Field

Example 8.1:

    (a) How many monitor units are needed to deliver 3 Gy to a depth of 7 cm using the Clinac-4 at 80 cm SAD, with a 6 x 12 cm field?

    (b) What is the SSD?

    (c) What is the field size on the skin?

(a) The monitor setting is found as follows:

$$T = \frac{D_p}{monitor\ factor \cdot TMR}$$

where T is the treatment time (in minutes or number of monitor units) and D_p is the prescription dose (in cGy or Gy).

The table of TMR values in Appendix D also displays the monitor factors for the Clinac-4. We must first find the equivalent square for a 6 x 12 cm field:

$$\frac{2\,(6\ x12)}{6+12} = \frac{144}{18} = 8.0\ cm$$

For an 8 cm square at a depth of 7 cm, the TMR is 0.819. The monitor factor is 0.984 cGy/ μ. Therefore, the treatment duration is:

$$T = \frac{(3.0\ Gy \cdot 100\ cGy/\ Gy)}{(0.819) \cdot (0.984\ cGy/\mu)} = 372\ \mu$$

(b) Since the source to axis distance is the sum of   the source to skin distance plus the skin to axis (isocenter) distance, then:

$$SSD = (SAD - depth) = (80 - 7)\ cm = 73\ cm$$

(c) The field size is always specified at the axis (isocenter). For SAD techniques, the field size on the skin can be found using the proportion for similar triangles which we used in Chapter 7, Section H:

$$\frac{Field\ edge\ at\ skin}{Field\ edge\ at\ isocenter} = \left(\frac{SSD}{SAD}\right)$$

Therefore:
(1) Field edge$_1$ at skin = 6 cm (73/80) = 5.48 cm
(2) Field edge$_2$ at skin = 12 cm (73/80) = 10.95 cm

Example 8.2:

Repeat the Example 8.1 using the Clinac-18
at 100 cm SAD.

(a) In Appendix E, we find the TMR and monitor factor from the same table for equivalent square 8 cm, TMR at 7.0 cm depth = 0.9, monitor factor = 0.981 cGy/μ. Thus the treatment duration for 3 Gy is:

$$T = \frac{D_0}{TMR \cdot monitor\ factor} = \frac{300cGy}{(0.900)(0.981\ cGy/\mu)} = 340\ \mu$$

(b) The SSD is 93 cm (100 cm - 7 cm)

(c) The field size on the skin is:

 (1) 6 cm (93/100) = 5.58 cm

 (2) 12 cm (93/100) = 11.16 cm

G.
Dose at Points Other Than the Isocenter

Calculating the dose at points other than the isocenter is not as simple as for SSD planning. With SSD planning, one simply sets up the proportion:

$$D_x / D_p = ddf_x / ddf_p$$

This procedure will not work for SAD planning. A four step procedure is required.

(1) Find the field size at the point of interest (X). Since the spec-ified field size is at isocenter (iso), where the prescription point usually lies, then the field size will be either larger or smaller at the new point, depending upon whether it is farther from or closer to the surface than the isocenter (iso). Again, the similar triangles proportion is used:

$$\frac{(equiv.\ square)_x}{(equiv.\ square)_{iso}} = \frac{source\ to\ (X)\ distance}{SAD}$$

The source to X distance = SAD - (depth of isocenter, which is depth from skin to isocenter) + (depth of X), where X is the point of interest, and the depths are measured from the skin. Notice that it is equal to SSD + (depth of X), so:

$$(equiv.\ square)_x = (equiv.\ square)_{iso} \cdot \left(\frac{SSD + depth\ of\ X}{SAD}\right)$$

(2) Look up the TMR for the field size found in Example 8.1 and depth of point X.

(3) Now adjust the monitor factors. Since the TMR you just looked up is valid with a monitor factor for a larger or small er field than the one actually being used, you must divide out the monitor factor for this field size (fs) and multiply in the correct one, for the field size at isocenter, i.e., corrected TMR:

$$\text{Corrected TMR} = \text{TMR (for field size at X)} \left(\frac{\text{monitor factor for field size at iso}}{\text{monitor factor for field size at X}}\right)$$

(4) Perform an inverse square law correction. This is a critical step because, in using the monitor factors valid at the isocenter (SAD), the entire table of TMR's becomes valid only at this distance. Since your point of interest is not at this distance (not at isocenter), you must multiply by the following:

$$\text{Inverse square factor (ISF)} = \left(\frac{SAD}{SSD + depth\ at\ X}\right)^2$$

Technically, this correction should be applied to the monitor factor (for field size at axis). Since this monitor factor already appears in the corrected TMR form from the previous step, we will apply it there.

$$TMR^* = corrected\ TMR \cdot (ISF) = corrected\ TMR \cdot \left(\frac{SAD}{SSD + depth\ at\ X}\right)^2$$

where TMR* is not a true TMR, but is the quantity which allows us to find the dose at the point of interest from D_{iso}, the dose at isocenter:

$$D_x = D_p \cdot \left(\frac{TMR^*}{TMR_{iso}}\right)$$

where TMR_{iso} is the tabulated TMR for the field size and depth at isocenter.

In the case where the prescription point is at point X ($D_p = D_x$), the dose at isocenter, D_{iso}, is given by:

$$D_{iso} = D_p \cdot \left(\frac{TMR_{iso}}{TMR^*}\right)$$

In addition, note that the inverse square correction is the most significant correction, and must never be omitted! (Even a 1 cm difference in the position of X will make a difference of 2% or more in dose.) The change of TMR with depth is the next most significant correction. Correcting the field size sometimes has a small effect.

Example 8.3:

For the case in Example 8.1, find D_{max}, and the dose at 13 cm depth.

Dose at d_{max} will occur at 1 cm depth. The field size there will be:

$$Equivalent\ square\ at\ 1\ cm\ = (equiv.\ square\ at\ iso)\left(\frac{SSD + 1\ cm}{SAD}\right)$$

$$= 8\ cm\ \left(\frac{74}{80}\right) = 7.4\ cm$$

Interpolating on the TMR table, we find that TMR (7.4 cm field) = 1.0, since we are at d_{max}, monitor factor (7.4 cm field) = 0.978 cGy/μ, and monitor factor (8 cm field) = 0.984 cGy/μ, so:

$$TMR*_{1\ cm} = (1.0)\left(\frac{80}{74}\right)^2\left(\frac{0.984}{0.978}\right) = 1.176$$

Thus the dose at d_{max} is:

$$D_{max} = D_p\left(\frac{TMR*}{TMR_p}\right) = 3\ Gy\left(\frac{1.176}{0.819}\right) = 4.31\ Gy$$

At 13 cm depth, the field size (equivalent square) is:

$$8\ cm\ \left(\frac{73 + 13}{80}\right) = 8.6\ cm$$

From the table, TMR (8.6 cm field, 13 cm depth) = 0.628, and monitor factor for 8.6 cm field = 0.988. So:

$$TMR* = 0.628\left(\frac{80}{73 + 13}\right)^2\left(\frac{0.984}{0.988}\right) = 0.541$$

And the dose at this point is:

$$D_{13} = 3\ Gy\left(\frac{0.541}{0.819}\right) = 1.98\ Gy$$

H.
Comparison of D_{max} for SSD and SAD Techniques

This is best done by example. Suppose we have a thin patient (14 cm thick) and wish to deliver 6 Gy at midline (these strange numbers were chosen in order to take advantage of the results of the previous examples).

We will first plan opposing fields using 79 cm SSD to treat this patient, delivering 3 Gy from each field to midline (7 cm). For a fair comparison, we must use the same field size we used in the previous examples. This is not an 8 cm equivalent square, except at 7 cm depth. At the surface, it is 8 cm (73/80) = 7.3 cm.

From the depth dose tables for CL-4, ddf (7.3 cm field, 7 cm depth) is equal to 0.711, monitor factor is 0.977, ddf (7.3 cm field, 13 cm depth) is 0.474, and ddf (d_{max}) is at 1.00.

$$D_1 = 3\,Gy\left(\frac{1.00}{0.711}\right) = 4.23\,Gy$$
$$D_7 = D_p = 3\,Gy$$
$$D_{13} = 3\,Gy\left(\frac{0.474}{0.711}\right) = 2\,Gy$$

To summarize the two techniques:

SAD Planning	**SSD Planning**
$D_1 = 4.31$ Gy	$D_1 = 4.23$ Gy
$D_7 = 3.00$ Gy	$D_7 = 3$ Gy
$D_{13} = 1.98$ Gy	$D_{13} = 2$ Gy

For opposing equally weighted fields, d_{max} for field #1 will be coincident with the 13 cm depth of field #2. To find the total dose at that point (d_{max} for field #1), we add $D_1 + D_{13}$ and compare it to the total dose of 6 Gy at the midline.

With SAD planning, $D_{max} = 6.29$ Gy
With SSD planning, $D_{max} = 6.23$ Gy

While these numbers are close, it is seen that **the subcutaneous dose is higher for SAD techniques than for SSD techniques**. In general this is true when the SSD and SAD are numerically about the same and treatment is done with the same therapy unit.

The reason for this is apparent when one expresses the SSD using the SAD technique (73 cm in this example). Since the SSD is smaller using the SAD technique, the depth dose percentages (if they are calculated) are smaller due to inverse square law correction (that is, when the patient is closer to the source, the dose drops off faster with depth). Therefore, by definition, the dose at d_{max} must be higher in order to achieve the same dose at the depth of interest.

I.
Calculation of Dose with Opposing Equally Weighted Fields

Often patients are treated with a pair of opposing fields, i.e., fields whose central rays coincide but which enter the patient from opposite directions.

Equal weight means that each of the two fields delivers the same dose to the prescription point (usually the isocenter). The fields are usually, but not necessarily, the same size.

The calculation of each field is done in the same way as already discussed. The total dose to any point is the sum of the doses received from each field.

Note that at the prescription point the total dose is twice the dose from a single field. At other points, the two doses must be calculated separately and then added.

The advantage of opposed fields with equal weight is that the dose distribution is almost homogeneous over the entire treated volume, except for the buildup regions. This effect, and the method of calculation, can be seen in an example:

Example 8.4:

> Two opposing equally weighted fields are used to treat a patient 14 cm thick. All the field parameters are the same as in examples 8.1 and 8.3, except that the total dose from one fraction both fields is 3 Gy at the iso-center (depth 7 cm).
> (a) How many monitor units are needed for each field?
> (b) What is the total dose at a depth of 1 cm from the side where field number 1 enters?
> (c) What is the total dose at a depth of 13 cm from the same side?

(a) Each field will contribute 1.5 Gy, half of what was calculated in Example 8.1. Thus, the treatment duration is halved to give 186 μ.
(b) The dose from field number 1 is at 1 cm depth; from Example 8.3, it must be half of 4.31 Gy, or 2.15 Gy. The dose from field number 2 is at 13 cm depth, and similarly must be half of 1.98 Gy, or 99 cGy.
(c) The two doses are merely reversed, so the total dose is also 3.14 Gy.

For any depths between 1 cm and 13 cm, calculation will show doses between 3 and 3.14 Gy. Thus, the maximum deviation from homogeneity, along the central ray, is 5%.

The homogeneity will be better for higher energy radiation, thinner body sections, and larger fields. The dose will be less uniform for lower energies, thicker sections, and smaller fields.

References

1. Johns, H.E. & Cunningham, J.R. *The Physics of Radiology*, 4th Edition, Charles C. Thomas, Springfield, 1983, pp. 341-342.
2. Holt, J.G., Laughlin, J.S., Moroney, J.P. "Extension of Concept of Tissue-Air Ratios (TAR) to High Energy X-Ray Beams," *Radiology* 96:437, 1970.
3. Khan, F.M., Sewchand, W., Lee, Z.J., Williamson, J.F. "Revision of Tissue-Maximum Ratio and Scatter-Maximum Ratio Concepts for Cobalt 60 and Higher Energy X-Ray Beams," *Medical Physics* 7:230, 1980.
4. Karzmark, C.J., Deubert, A., Loevinger, R. "Tissue-Phantom Ratios: An Aid to Treatment Planning," *Br J Radiol* 38:158, 1965.
5. AAPM Task Group 21. "A Protocol for the Determination of Absorbed Dose from High-Energy Photon and Electron Beams," *Med Phys* 10(6), pp. 741-771, 1983.
6. *Radiation Dosimetry: X-Rays and Gamma Rays with Maximum Phantom Energies Between 0.6 and 50 MeV*, Report 14, International Commission on Radiation Units and Measurements, Washington, D.C., 1969, Appendix B.

Weighted Radiation Fields

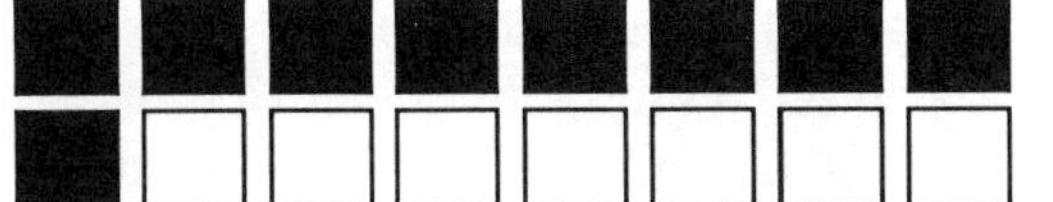

9

A. Opposing Weighted Fields
B. Multiple Weighted Fields - Cycle Time
C. Calculating Timer or Integrator Settings With Multiple
   Weighted Fields

Field weights are used differently in SAD planning than in SSD planning. In SSD planning, the relative weights of two or more fields is the ratio of the doses delivered by each field to its own depth of maximum dose (d_{max}). For example, if field number one delivers 2 Gy to its d_{max} and field number two delivers 1.5 Gy to its d_{max} (not considering the dose from field 1 to d_{max} of field 2, and vice versa), then the fields will have relative weights 1.0 to 0.75 (or 100 to 75 on a percentage basis). Of course, since weights are relative, we could also call these weights 200 to 150, or 400 to 300, as long as the ratio is the same. For reasons explained later, you should always have at least one field with a weight of 1.00 (or 100). It would be sufficient in the above example to assign a weight of 1.0 to field number two, giving a weight of 1.33 to field number one.

In SAD planning, field weights are calculated at the axis, rather than at buildup. This will give the same result as above only when the skin to axis distance is the same for all fields involved. This is extremely unlikely unless there are only two opposing fields and the prescription point is at mid-patient.

A.
Opposing Weighted Fields

Since we have already considered equally weighted opposing ports in some detail, we will now consider weights of 2:1 and greater.

Example 9.1:

As an example of a SSD planning and of a resulting dose distribution, calculate a central ray dose profile for a patient (20 cm thick) treated with opposing 10 x 10 cm 4 MV x-ray beams. The weight of beam 1 is to be twice that of beam 2, and a total dose of 60 Gy is to be delivered to a depth of 1 cm on the side nearest beam 1. Use 79 cm SSD.

We shall calculate the dose in 3 cm increments along the central ray; i.e., at 1, 4, 7, 10, 13, 16 and 19 cm. For this we shall need the following data from the 4 MV depth dose table:

$$ddf_1 = 1.00$$
$$ddf_4 = 0.861$$
$$ddf_7 = 0.724$$
$$ddf_{10} = 0.601$$
$$ddf_{13} = 0.496$$
$$ddf_{16} = 0.400$$
$$ddf_{19} = 0.327$$
$$\text{monitor factor} = 1.00$$

The dose specified for d_{max} of beam number 1 is 60 Gy total. How much of this is to come from each field?

Call the points listed above points A, B, C, D, E, F, and G corresponding to depth of 1, 4, 7, 10, 13, 16, and 19 cm from the side at which beam 1 enters. Point A is at d_{max} for field 1 (f_1), and point G is at d_{max} for field 2 (f_2). We can write two equations for this problem:

(1) Dose at A from (f_1) = 2 x Dose at G from (f_2), i.e., $D_1 f_1 = 2D_1 (f_2)$

(2) $D_1 f_1 + D_{19} f_2 = 60$ Gy; i.e., $D_1 (f_1) \times ddf_1 + D_1 (f_2) \times ddf_{19} = 60$ Gy

Substituting the first equation into the first term of the second equation gives:

$$2D_1 (f_2) \times ddf_1 + D_1 (f_2) \times ddf_{19} = 60 \, Gy$$

which can be rewritten as:

$$D_1 (f_2) \times (2ddf_1 + ddf_{19}) = 60 \, Gy$$

and finally:

$$D_1\left(f_2\right)=\frac{60\,Gy}{2ddf_1+ddf_{19}}=\frac{60\,Gy}{2.327}=25.78\,Gy$$

and thus:

$$D_1\left(f_1\right)\;=\;2\;x\,25.78\,Gy\;=\;51.56\,Gy$$

We are now prepared to calculate the profile, knowing the doses of points A - G:

A= D_1 (f$_1$) ddf$_1$ + D_1 (f$_2$) ddf$_{19}$ = 51.56 x 1.00 + 25.78 x 0.327 = 60 Gy
B= D_1 (f$_1$) ddf$_4$ + D_1 (f$_2$) ddf$_{16}$ = 51.56 x 0.861 + 2578 x 0.400 = 54.71 Gy
C= D_1 (f$_1$) ddf$_7$ + D_1 (f$_2$) ddf$_{13}$ = 51.56 x 0.724 + 2578 x 0.496 = 50.12 Gy
D= D_1 (f$_1$ ddf$_{10}$ + D_1 (f$_1$) ddf$_{10}$ = 51.56 x 0.601 + 2578 x 0.601 = 46.48 Gy
E= D_1 (f$_1$) ddf$_{13}$ + D_1 (f$_2$) ddf$_7$ = 51.56 x 0.496 + 2578 x 0.724 = 44.24 Gy
F= D_1 (f$_1$) ddf$_{16}$ + D_1 (f$_2$) ddf$_4$ = 51.56 x 0.400 + 2578 x 0.861 = 42.82 Gy
G= D_1 (f$_1$) ddf$_{19}$ + D_1 (f$_2$) ddf$_1$ = 51.56 x 0.327 + 2578 x 1.00 = 42.64 Gy

One can go through the same procedure with weight ratios of 3:1:

D_1 (f$_1$) = 3D_1 (f$_2$)
D_1 (f$_1$) + D_{19} (f$_2$) = 60 Gy = 3D_1 (f$_2$) + D_1 (f$_2$) ddf$_{19}$
D_1 (f$_2$) = 60 Gy / (3 + ddf$_{19}$) = 60 Gy / 3.327 = 18.03 Gy
D_1 (f$_1$) = 3D_1 (f$_2$) = 3 x 18.03 Gy = 54.10 Gy

whereupon the same point by point calculations as above gives dose to A, 60 Gy; dose to B, 53.79 Gy; dose to C, 48.11 Gy; dose to D, 43.35 Gy; dose to E, 39.89 Gy; dose to F, 37.16 Gy; and dose to G, 35.72 Gy.

These results are plotted in Figure 9.1, along with dose profiles for equally weighted fields, and a profile with f$_2$ weighted zero (treatment from one side only).

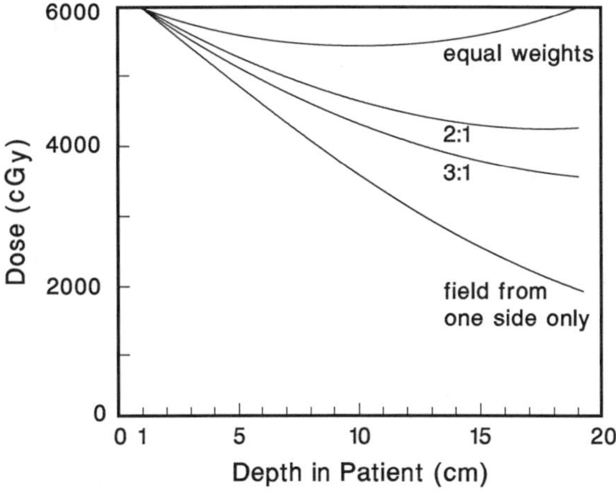

Figure 9.1. Graphical presentation of results of Example 9.1, along with results for equally weighted opposing field technique and treatment with a single field from one side only.

Examination of the curves in Figure 9.1 leads you to conclude that the use of opposing fields of unequal weight can be made to simulate a single field from one side of a higher energy. For example, the curve for 3:1 weighting looks like a single field depth dose curve, except for the failure to "drop off" sufficiently at depths greater than 10 cm.

If this is true, why should we spend huge sums of money for high energy treatment units? Why not buy a cobalt unit and use clever weighting of opposing fields to simulate the higher energy?

The answer is, of course, that you can simulate only single field distributions for higher energy. There is no way to use a cobalt-60 unit to duplicate the dose profile due to opposing 10MV fields of the same size; and single field treatment of deep lesions is rarely ever used with any energy.

There are occasions, however, when you will want to use such a scheme to treat bilaterally with a moderate dose while delivering a high dose to one side only.

B.
Multiple Weighted Fields - Cycle Time

There will be many situations where more than two fields are required to adequately treat a tumor, and it may be that no two fields are opposing, and no two fields have the same weight. Isodose summation is mandatory in such cases. Even so, it is frighteningly easy to err in the calculation of timer or monitor settings in such complicated cases. This is particularly true when you have the options of SSD or SAD planning, since the concept of weights is different for these two techniques. What you need to follow is a cookbook scheme to avoid such systematic error. It also pays to have someone independently check the calculations.

In the following approach, the term "cycle time" will be used. This concept is necessary because sometimes not all the fields involved are treated on the same day. From a radiobiological standpoint, it is nearly always a good idea to do so, but sometimes it is not practical.[1] In such cases, a greater target volume dose may be accomplished in one fraction day than in the next, because of the different number or weights of the fields involved on those two days. Nevertheless, the aim is for the daily dose to "average out" to a given prescription dose; for example, 2 Gy per fraction.

Cycle time is the smallest number of days over which this averaging can be accurately done. For example, suppose two fields are involved. One is weighted 1.0 and is treated every day. The second is weighted 0.2 and is treated every other day. On those days when only field one is used, somewhat less than the average prescription dose is delivered. On those days when both fields are treated, somewhat more than the average prescription dose is delivered. If an average is taken every other treatment day, however, the result will be the same as if the average was taken over the entire duration of the treatment program. The cycle time in this case is two days.

It is easy to fall into the trap of assuming that the cycle time is the number of days during which each involved field has been treated at least once. This is usually, but not always, true.

Consider this hypothetical case. Three fields are to be used to deliver a total of 45 Gy in 18 fractions to a specified point (or more appropriately, the boundary of a specified volume).   The three fields have weights of 1 : 2/9 : 1/6 (or 100 : 22.2 : 16.7). It is decided to use field number one every fraction, delivering 1.8 Gy to the prescription point. Field two will be used every second treatment day, each time for 80 cGy; and field three will be used every third treatment day, each time for 90 cGy. This situation is outlined in Table 9.1.

Table 9.1:

Fraction Day	cGy Field 1	cGy Field 2	cGy Field 3	cGy this fraction	Accumulated Gy
1	180	--	--	180	1.80
2	180	80	--	260	4.40
3	180	--	90	270	7.10
4	180	80	--	260	9.70
5	180	--	--	180	11.50
6	180	80	90	350	15.00
7	180	--	--	180	16.80
8	180	80	--	260	19.40
9	180	--	90	270	22.10
10	180	80	--	260	24.70
11	180	--	--	180	26.50
12	180	80	90	350	30.00
13	180	--	--	180	31.80
14	180	80	--	260	34.40
15	180	--	90	270	37.10
16	180	80	--	260	39.70
17	180	--	--	180	41.50
18	180	80	90	350	45.00

You see from this table that over the entire 18 fraction days the accumulated dose is 45 Gy, so the average fraction is 45 Gy/ 18 fractions = 2.5 Gy/fraction.

You also see that all fields have been treated at least once over a time period of the first three days. This is not the cycle time. The accumulated dose after three days is 7.1 Gy. Thus the average dose per fraction is 7.1 Gy/3 fractions = 2.37 Gy/fraction.

The cycle time in this example is six days. Every six days, 15 Gy has accumulated, so the average dose per fraction is 15 Gy/6 fractions = 2.5 Gy/fraction, which is the same as the average taken over the entire program.

You should avoid complicated fractionation schedules such as this. It should always be feasible to arrange the schedule so that the cycle time coincides with the number of days necessary to treat all fields at least once. If there is any doubt, a good procedure is to chart out the entire program as was done in Table 9.1.

C.
Calculating Timer or Integrator Settings With Multiple Weighted Fields

In the following example it is assumed that:
(a) The total dose and total number of fractions is known (note: this is the prescription).
(b) An isodose summation has been performed. The isodose value which best bounds the target volume has been selected by the therapist, physicist, or dosimetrist.
(c) The weights of all involved fields are known (if this were not true, no isodose summation would have been possible).
(d) A time schedule has been arranged for all involved fields if they are not all to be treated each fraction day, and the cycle time has been determined.

The first question is what do the values of the isodose lines represent? For example, an isodose line having a value of 165% (or 1.65) may surround the target volume. 165% of what?

These values are interpreted differently for SSD and SAD planning. In the SSD case, 165 % means that "all points on this line receive 165% as much dose as is given by any 100 weight field to its own normalizing point (or d_{max} on the central ray)." This is why we insisted earlier that at least one field should have a weight of 100 (or 1.0).

In the SAD case, the isodose line passing through the axis has a value equal to the sum of all fields involved. For example, if three fields weighted 100, 40, and 15 are used isocentrically, the value of the isodose line which passes through the axis will be 155% (or 1.55). All other isodose lines in the summation are relative to this. For example, if 3 Gy is absorbed at the axis (1.55 line), then the dose on the 120% (1.2) line will be:

$$\frac{1.2}{1.55} \times 3 \, Gy = 2.32 \, Gy$$

Of course, this relative value property of isodose lines in the summation is true for SSD patterns as well. Some planners choose other normalizations such as 100% to the isocenter, but relative calculation will still be done as above.

The promised cookbook approach to determining timer or integrator settings follows. **For SSD planning the procedure is as follows:**

(a) Multiply the average dose per fraction times the number of fraction days in the cycle time, to obtain the total dose per cycle time.

(b) Divide this dose per cycle time by the decimal value of the isodose line which has been selected for the prescription dose (i.e., if the line has a value of 160%, divide by 1.6). Call the result "100 weight dose per cycle."

(c) Find any field which has an assigned weight of 100 (or 1.0) and determine the number of times it will be applied per cycle.

(d) Divide this number into the result of step (b), the 100 weight dose per cycle.

(e) The result is the dose given by this 100 weight field to its own normalization point, per fraction. The same will be true for any other field with a weight of 100.

(f) For any field whose weight is not 100, multiply the weight of the field (decimal value) times the 100 weight dose per cycle from step (b) and divide this by the number of fractions per cycle for this field. The result is the dose per fraction given by this field to its own normalization point.

(g) For each field, find the treatment duration as outlined in the section on single field; i.e., divide the dose by CAL, (or CAL x BF and/or f, depending on the type of calibration sheet).

For SAD planning, the procedure is as follows:

(a) Find the prescription dose per cycle time as before, multiplying average dose per fraction times number of fraction days per cycle.

(b) Calculate the cycle dose at the isocenter, by dividing the decimal value of the selected isodose line into the value of the isocenter isodose line (which is, recall, equal to the sum of all weights), and multiplying this ratio times the result of step (a), dose per cycle time at the prescription time.

(c) For any field, divide its weight by the isodose value at isocen
ter (for example, if the isocenter isodose line is 160 and the
weight is 30, divide 30 / 160, or .3 / 1.6). Multiply this ratio
times the result of step (b), cycle dose at isocenter.
(d) Divide this result by the number of times this field is used per
cycle time. The answer is the dose given to the isocenter per
fraction by this field.
(e) To obtain treatment duration, divide this result by CAL and
TMR (or TAR, or TPR, depending on calibration type). For
this treatment duration it is necessary to know the skin to isocenter distance for each field in question.

Example 9.2:

Figure 9.2 shows the set-up for a patient who is to receive 60 Gy in 30 fractions using Clinac-4 fields at 79
cm SSD. Calculate the integrator settings for the three
fields. Field one and two are treated on day one, fields
one and three on day two, and fields one and two on
day three, and so on.

*Figure 9.2. Three
fields set-up.*

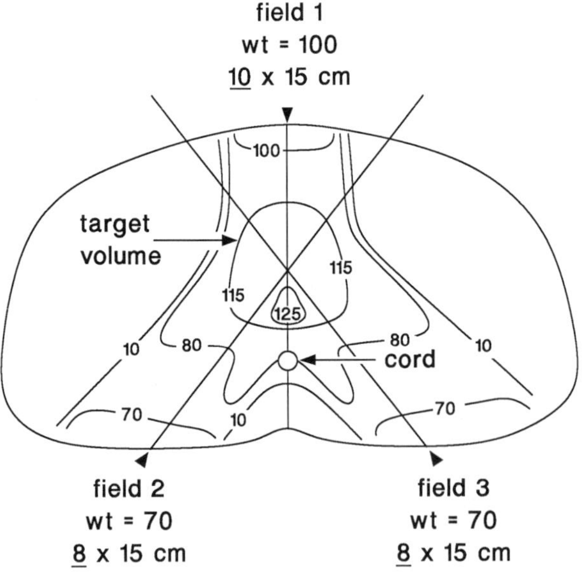

Assume the 115% line encompasses the target volume, and
the prescription dose pertains to this line. Step (a) in the recipe:
the average dose per fraction is 60 Gy / 30 fractions = 2 Gy per
fraction. The cycle time is two days, so the total dose per cycle

is 4 Gy. Step (b): 100 weight dose per cycle = 4 Gy / 1.15 = 3.48 Gy. Steps (c, d, e): for field 1, which has weight 100 and is treated twice per cycle, the maximum dose per fraction is 3.48 Gy / 2 = 1.74 Gy. Step (f): for field 2 or 3, (weight 70, one time each per cycle):

$$dose\ at\ d_{max}\ per\ fraction\ = \frac{0.7 \times 3.48\ Gy}{1\ application} = 2.44\ Gy\ per\ application$$

Step (g): treatment durations:

$$field\ 1,\ T = \frac{1.74\ Gy}{1.01\ cGy/\mu} = 172\ \mu$$

$$fields\ 2\ and\ 3,\ T = \frac{2.44\ Gy}{1.002\ cGy/\mu} = 244\ \mu$$

(1.01 cGy /μ and 1.002 cGy /μ are the monitor factors for Cl-4 fields whose equivalent squares are 12.0 cm and 10.4 cm, corresponding to 10 x 15 cm and 8 x 15 cm fields.) Note that field size factor is normalized to unity for a 10 x 10 cm field.

Example 9.3:

> For this same patient, estimate the total dose to the anterior portion of the spinal cord, and the maximum delivered dose. From Figure 9.2, the isodose line at the anterior portion of the cord has a value of 80%. The dose will be given by:

$$\frac{dose\ to\ cord}{80} = \frac{dose\ to\ target\ volume}{115}$$

So:

$$dose\ to\ cord = 60\ Gy \left(\frac{80}{115}\right) = 41.74\ Gy$$

The maximum isodose value in the summation is 125%, so the dose there is:

$$maximum\ dose = \frac{125 \times 60\ Gy}{115} = 65.22\ Gy$$

Example 9.4:

Figure 9.3 shows the treatment plan of a patient who is to receive 50 Gy in 20 fractions to the target volume outlined by the 240% line. Four fields are used isocentrically. Fields 1 and 3 are treated each fraction day, field 2 is treated every second fraction day, and field 4 is treated every fourth fraction day. Calculate monitor settings, assuming these are Clinac-4 fields.

Figure 9.3. Four fields set-up.

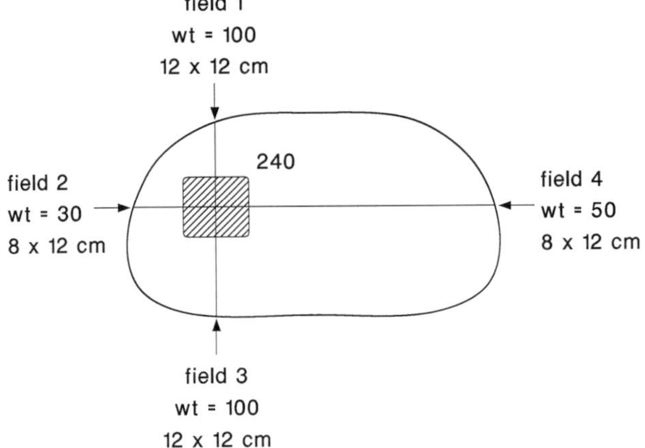

Step (a):

$$average\ dose\ per\ fraction = \frac{50\ Gy}{20\ fractions} = 2.5\ Gy/fraction$$

Cycle time is 4 fractions. Thus:

$$prescription\ dose\ per\ cycle\ time = 2.5\ Gy \times 4 = 10\ Gy$$

Step (b): The isodose value at the isocenter will equal the sum of all weights, which is 280. Thus:

$$the\ dose\ per\ cycle\ at\ isocenter = \frac{280}{240}(10\ Gy) = 11.67\ Gy$$

Step (c): The dose to the isocenter from field one (weight 100, 4 times per cycle) will be:

$$\frac{100}{280}(11.67)/4\ applications = 1.04\ Gy\,/\,application$$

Similarly for field 3, the dose to the isocenter from field 2 (weight 50, 2 times per cycle) will be:

$$\frac{50}{280}(11.67)/2\ applications = 1.04\ Gy\,/\,application$$

And to the isocenter dose from field 4 (weight 30, 1 time per cycle) will be:

$$\frac{30}{280}(11.67) / 1 \; application = 1.25 \; Gy / application$$

Step (e): To find treatment durations, we need not only the field size factors for each field, but also the TMR for the skin to axis distance for each field. From the TMR sheet:

Field #	1	2	3	4
Field Size Factor	1.010	0.996	1.010	0.996
TMR	0.813	0.454	0.813	0.731

(The equivalent square for fields 2 and 4 is 9.6 cm^2.)

$$for \; fields \; 1 \; and \; 3, \quad T = \frac{1.04 \; Gy}{(.813) \times (1.01 \; cGy/\mu)} = 127 \; \mu$$

$$for \; field \; 2, \quad T = \frac{1.04 \; Gy}{(.454) \times (.996 \; cGy/\mu)} = 230 \; \mu$$

$$for \; field \; 4, \quad T = \frac{1.25 \; Gy}{(.731) \times (.996) \; cGy/\mu} = 172 \; \mu$$

Reference

1. Wilson, C.S. & Hall, E.J. "On the Advisability of Treating All Fields at Each Radiotherapy Session," *Radiology* 98:419, 1971.

Isodose Curves for Single and Multiple Fields

10

A. Correction for Sloping Surface or Non-Perpendicular Entry
B. Interpolating an Isodose Distribution for an Intermediate Field Size
C. Adjusting an Isodose Distribution for a Weighted Field
D. Isodose Summation by the Superposition Method
E. Past-Pointing
F. Two-Field Isodose Summations in SSD Planning
G. Multiple Opposing Pairs in SSD Planning
H. Three-Field Technique in SSD Planning
I. Isodose Curves for SAD Planning
J. Isodose Summation Using SAD Type Isodose Curves
K. Isodose Summation by Computer

Many treatment decisions and calculations are based on treatment plans which consist of isodose distribution superimposed on patient cross-sections. These plans are now usually produced by a computerized treatment planning system. The last section of this chapter discusses why it is valuable to be able to produce isodose distributions by hand from sets of isodose curves from single fields.

Single field isodose distributions are measured under "ideal" conditions; i.e., perpendicular entry through a flat surface into a perfectly homogeneous medium which is semi-infinite. With the exception of perpendicular entry, none of these ideal conditions is encountered in patient treatment.

It is therefore necessary to know how to correct for the lack of one or more of the above conditions, as well as how to combine isodoses from more than one field. The basic techniques are covered in this chapter.

A.
Correction for Sloping Surface or Non-Perpendicular Entry

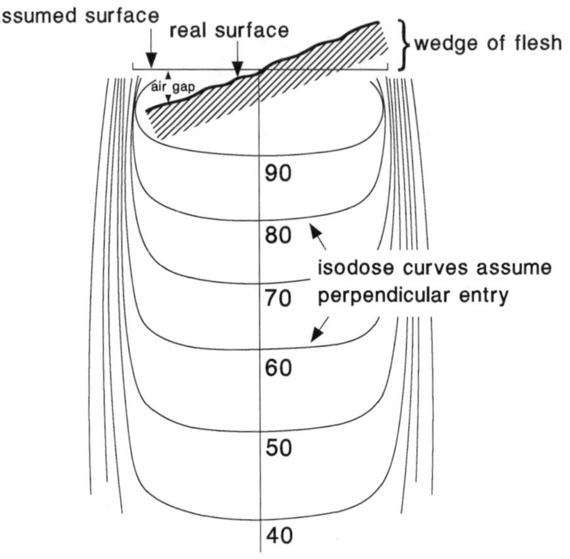

Figure 10.1. Standard single field isodose distribution of a perpendicular beam through a flat surface. The medium is assumed to be homogeneous.

Refer to Figure 10.1. A standard isodose distribution is placed on a sloping body part so that the central ray entry point is at the surface. Since the supposed surface is perpendicular to the central ray, whereas the skin surface is not, there is an air gap on one side of the field and a wedge of flesh on the other, neither of which is accounted for in the position of the isodose curves.

One solution, much used in the days of primarily orthovoltage "deep therapy," was to add sufficient bolus at the surface to make it flat and perpendicular to the central ray. As discussed earlier, this causes the tissue maximum dose to fall near the skin surface and is unacceptable with linear accelerators, since no advantage is taken of skin sparing.

There are a number of mathematical approaches to the problem of non-perpendicular entry, all of which are somewhat involved and time consuming, thus suited to computer planning.[1,2,3,4] If you have to calculate corrections by hand, you would do few isodose summations, since nearly all skin surfaces are sloping, requiring a tedious calculation.

A reasonably easy method of correction using hand calculation is the isodose shift method. This involves the following steps:

(a) Place the patient contour over a standard isodose distribution
   for the treatment unit and field size in question, in such a way

that the real and supposed surfaces coincide at the central ray (Figure 10.2).

(b) Draw in a divergent ray pattern, with rays at several intervals spanning the full primary portion of the field (such a pattern should already be on hand in the dosimetry room).

(c) Measure the distances between the assumed surface of the isodose distribution and the real surface of the patient, along the diverging rays. Call these distances Δ_1, Δ_2, etc. See Figure 10.2 for a more detailed illustration.

(d) Shift all points of intersection between isodose lines and diverging rays by an amount $k\Delta$, where Δ is the gap distance for that divergent ray, and k values are given in Table 10.1. (For example, k for a cobalt-60 at 80 cm SSD is 0.7, so if Δ on a given line is 12 mm, the shift would be 0.7 x 12 mm = 8 mm.) The direction of shift is shown in Figure 10.2; if the gap is air, shift the points down; if the gap is tissue, shift the points up.

(e) Join the shifted points with a smooth line. These are the new positions of the isodose curves. Allow them to join the old isodose curves in the penumbra region. The direction of shift is shown in Figure 10.2; the gap is air.

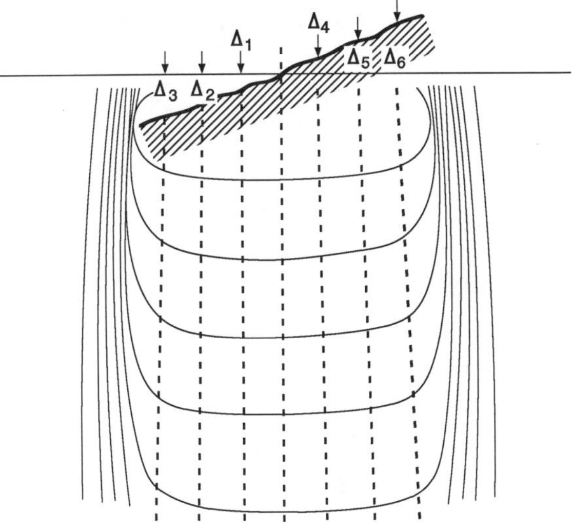

Figure 10.2. Patient contour, isodose distribution, and diverging ray pattern in overlay. Δ_1, Δ_2, and Δ_3 are air gaps measured along the diverging rays between the assumed surface of the isodose distribution and the true surface. Δ_4, Δ_5, and Δ_6 are the corresponding flesh gaps on the other side of the field.

While this sounds like a lengthy procedure, with a little practice an entire isodose distribution can be so shifted within a few minutes (see Figure 10.3).

The value of k usually depends not only on the photon energy, but on SSD, field size, and depth. The values given in Table 10.1 are for typical field sizes (10 x 10 cm to 20 x 20 cm) and for

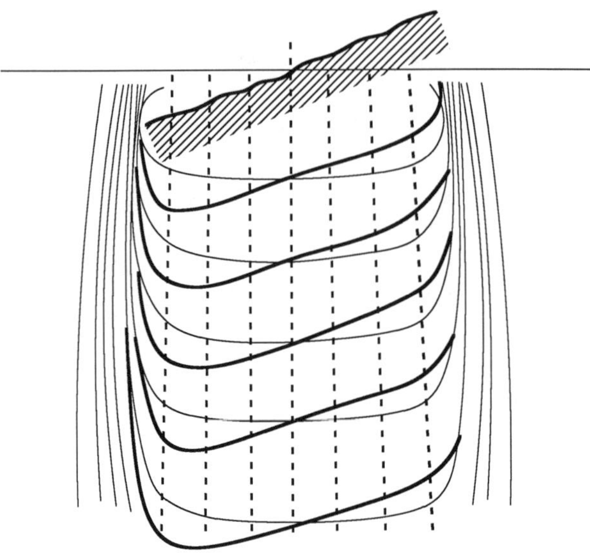

SSD of 80 to 100 cm.[5,6] If very nonstandard SSD's are used, chances are you will have no recorded isodose distributions to shift.

Table 10.1. Shift factor k for various photon energies.

Photon Energy	k
150 kV - 1 MV	0.8
1 MV - 5 MV	0.7
Cobalt-60	0.75
5 MV - 15 MV	0.6
15 MV - 30 MV	0.5
greater than 30 MV	0.4

B.
Interpolating an Isodose Distribution for an Intermediate Field Size

If you perform isodose summations by hand, then you must rely on isodose distributions on file for that machine. It is unlikely that there will be a "complete" inventory. For example, if you decide you need a 9 x 15 cm isodose map, you may find in the file an 8 x 15 cm and a 10 x 15 cm, but no 9 x 15 cm map.

At this point, many people would either rationalize that the use of the 10 x 15 cm field would be clinically expedient or

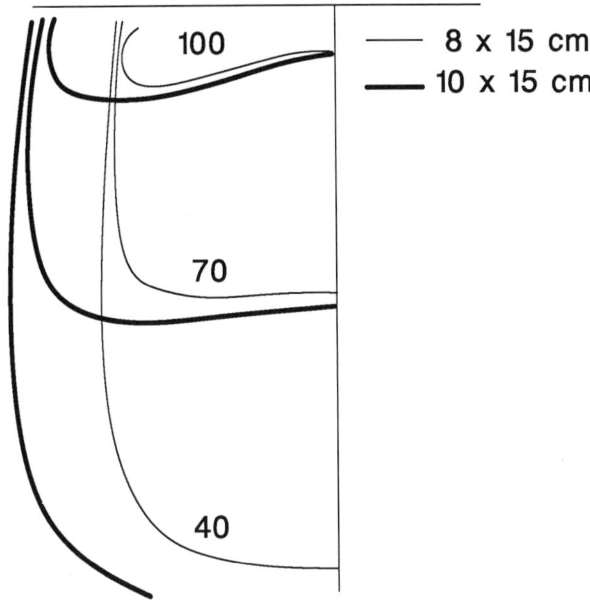

Figure 10.4. The 100%, 70%, and 40% isodose lines for 8 x 15 cm and 10 x 15 cm fields.

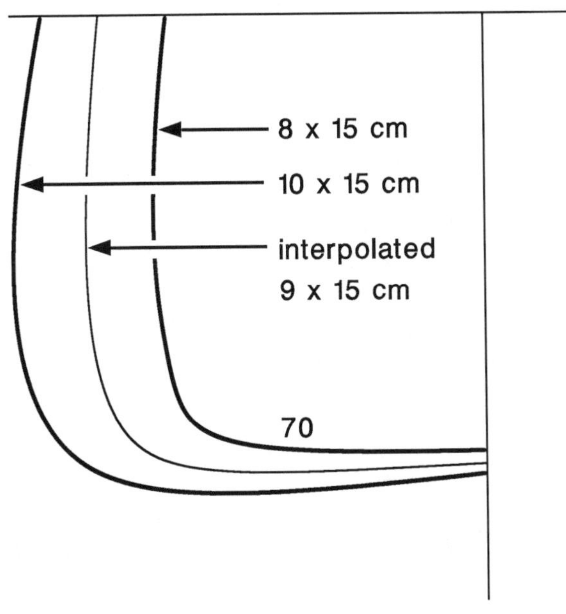

Figure 10.5. Interpolated isodose line for 9 x 15 cm field using 8 x 15 cm and 10 x 15 cm fields.

would go ahead and use the 9 x 15 cm field on the patient, failing to do an isodose summation.

A third alternative would be to use the isodose maps for the two closest field sizes (in the above example, 8 x 15 cm and 10 x 15 cm) and then do an analog interpolation to obtain the isodose map for the desired field size.

It is difficult to overlay two complete isodose maps on a light box and try to interpolate between them. One procedure which takes a little more time but is much easier on the eyes is to trace three isodose lines widely separated in value - for example, the 100%, 70%, and 40% - from each of the two distributions, and overlay the copied lines on a light box, being sure that the surface lines and central ray coincide.

Then, for each isodose line, trace the interpolated line representing the 9 x 15 cm field. It will be halfway between the isodose lines for the 8 x 15 cm field and the 10 x 15 cm field.

Now, do this procedure for other lines at 90%, 60%, and 30% dose. Then interpolate the remaining lines for the 80%, 50%, 20% and 10% values (these last two will be in the penumbra only).

The last step is to overlay the interpolated lines for the 9 x 15 cm field and transfer them to the same sheet, again being careful to align the surface and central ray lines.

For an unmodified field, all the forgoing steps can be done for half the field, since the curves you have are probably symmetrical around the central ray. Now you can fold the paper along the central ray and trace off the opposite side of the field.

If done carefully, this yields an acceptable interpolated field size isodose map.

If the first dimension of the desired field is the same as the first dimensions of two fields for which you have isodose curves, the interpolation is much easier and can be done in one step, since the penumbras of the two fields will very nearly match. For example, if you have isodose maps for 10 x 10 cm fields and 10 x 20 cm fields, and require one for a 10 x 15 cm field, then you need only interpolate in the full primary portion of the field and make the penumbra match that of either field for which you have curves. (The penumbras are not really the same, but usually the interpolated value will not vary much more than the width of your pencil lead, except for the 10% line.)

C.
Adjusting an Isodose Distribution for a Weighted Field

All isodose distributions which you have on file will have an assumed weight of 100. If you wish to do a summation in which one or more fields has a weight other than 100, you must modify the isodose distribution before summation.

If the new weight is 50, your procedure is simply to change the values of the already existing isodose curve. Where 100% becomes 50%, 80% becomes 40%, 60% becomes 30%, and so on.

(Note: on the finished single field distribution, you want isodose values which are multiples of 10. Otherwise, the summation procedure which follows becomes very difficult and confusing.)

If the new weight is, say, 30, then you must again interpolate. For example, on the old distribution the 100% line becomes the 30% line, which you can transfer directly; but the 90% line becomes the 27% line, which you do not want. The 70% line becomes the 21% line, and the 60% line becomes the 18% line, two lines that you also do not want. What you want is the 20% line, which you must obtain by interpolation between the 21% (70%) and 18% (60%) lines.

D.
Isodose Summation by the Superposition Method

Let us assume that you wish to obtain an isodose summation map in a clinical situation where two fields are being used. Also assume that you have isodose distributions for the two fields and that you have adjusted their weights, if this was necessary. You also have obtained a cross sectional contour map of the patient at the level of the central rays, and have marked within it the target volume and possibly some constraints, such as the eyes or spinal cord, etc.

Now you overlay the patient contour and one of the individual isodose distributions on a light box in such a way that the beam is directed as you desire (angle and point of entry), and the point where the central ray meets the supposed surface is also the point where it meets the real surface. You now modify this distribution for skin curvature using the isodose shift method of Chapter 10, Section A.

Do the same for the other field. You will now have modified isodose curves from two fields within the patient contour, forming a large number of intersecting lines. See Figure 10.6. Looking just below and to the right of the crossing point of the two central rays, you will see in Figure 10.6 a point of intersection of the 60% line of field one and the 60% line of field two. The summed value at this point is 120%.

Now look around for other intersections whose summed value is 120%. One such point is where these same two lines cross above and to the left of the central rays. Other intersection points are the four points of intersection of the 50% and 70% lines, and four points of intersection of 40% with 80% lines. These points have been marked on Figure 10.6 with tiny circles. Other possibilities would be of intersections of 30% with 90% lines, and

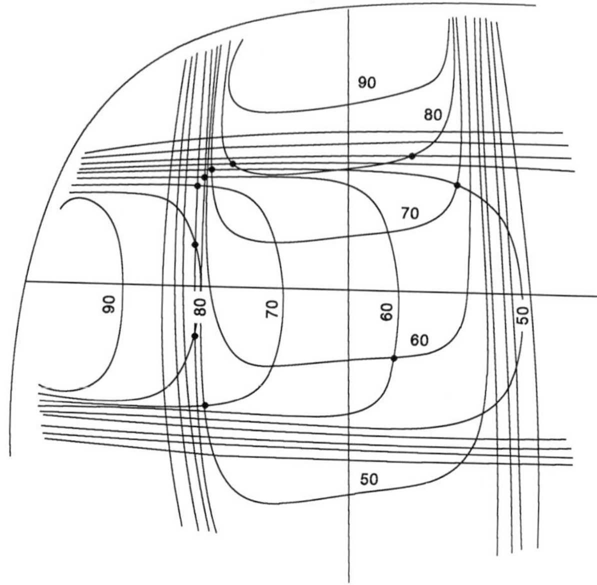

Figure 10.6. Schematic of procedure of an isodose summation of two fields.

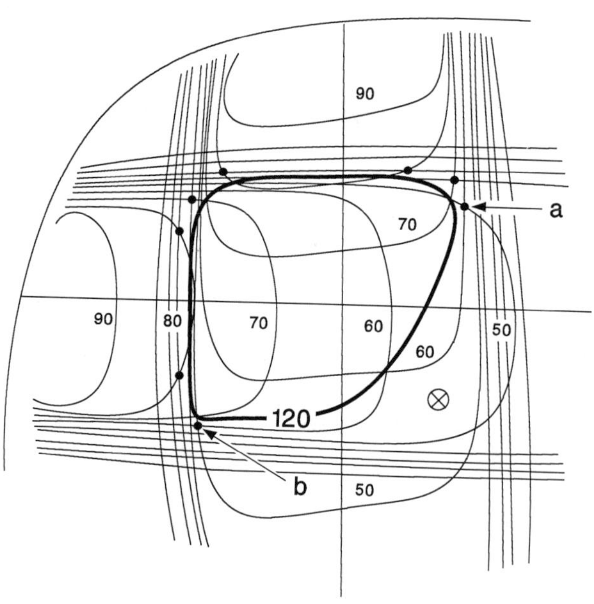

Figure 10.7. Schematic of 120% isodose line of two fields.

20% with 100% lines, but these do not occur in this particular case.

The summed 120% line is now obtained by connecting all these intersections with a smooth curve, as in Figure 10.7. Also on this figure, note that intersections have been marked which will yield summed 130% and 110% lines.

The small x in the lower right quadrant represents the 110% line, except there is no intersection here. This is the position where the values from each of the two fields is 55%. Sometimes it is necessary (as in this case) to use such points to determine where a summation line belongs, when there is a great separation between intersection points, (e.g., the points marked (a) and (b) in Figure 10.7).

Proceeding in this way, you obtain summed curves from 140% down to 20%, as shown in Figure 10.8.

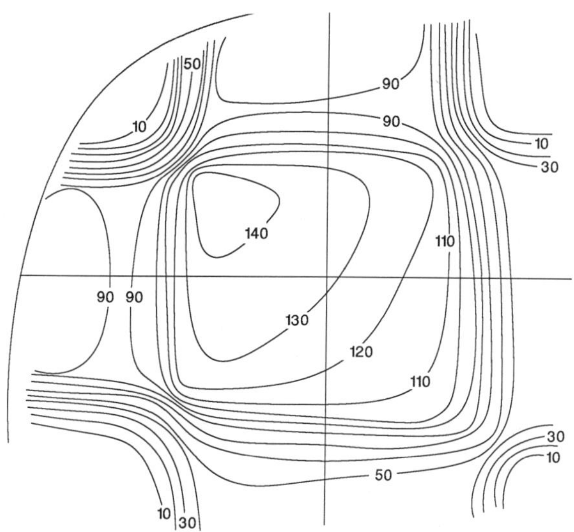

Figure 10.8. Schematic of final summation of all isodose lines of two fields.

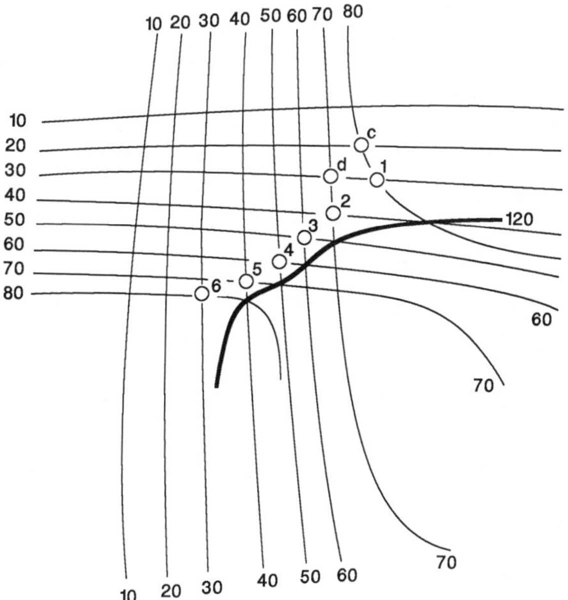

Figure 10.9. Schematic for intersection yielding a summation value of 120%.

A simple technique for locating points of intersection yielding summation values for the same isodose line is illustrated in Figure 10.9. This assumes that there are no isodose lines from the individual fields other than those which are multiples of 10, and that all of these lines are present.

Figure 10.9 is an enlargement of a small section of Figure 10.7 from the upper left quadrant. At this point, the 120% line has been drawn, and you are looking for the intersections yielding a summation value of 110%. You have located point (1), intersection of field 1 (80%) with field 2 (30%).

You now look for the nearest intersection which cannot be reached along an already existing single line. This is obviously point 2. Points (c) and (d) are nearer, but they are connected to point (1) by an existing line.

You do not have to stop and check the values of the lines whose intersection is point (2) in order to determine if the summation value is the same as point (1). You may simply draw the summation curve from point (1) to point (2); and from there to points (3), (4), (5), etc.

Again, this technique will work only if all pertinent lines are present which are multiples of 10, and no other lines are present in the individual field isodose summations.

Suppose there are three or more fields to sum, rather than two. Do not attempt to sum with more than two sets of curves. You may do this in order to find dose values at individual points, but to attempt to obtain summed curves from more than two distributions at once would be folly. (You should try it once, however, to satisfy yourself of this.)

When more than two fields are used, you must sum in pairs, then sum the summations, so that you are always dealing with no more than two distributions at one time. This involves extra time (and extra paper), but it will lead to a successful conclusion.

E.
Past-Pointing

Now we take a critical look at the results of our efforts and find an undesirable isodose distribution. In Figure 10.8, the "hottest" isodose curves (140, 130, 120) form concentric candy drop shapes which are much smaller than the field sizes used to form them. Furthermore, if the two fields used were "aimed" at the target volume, these high dose areas would likely miss the target and occur in surrounding tissue. If we wish these "hot spots" to occur in the target volume, we must direct the central rays so that they cross below or past the target. This is a general principle called **past pointing**.

When two nonparallel opposed fields are used, their central rays must cross below the center of the target volume.

Unfortunately, there is no formula to help you determine how far to past point. This depends on field size, depth, angle between beams, skin curvature, and type of radiation. You must rely on a combination of experience and trial and error. Nevertheless, if you position the two individual field isodose maps briefly on the contour and check the summed dose values at a few points, even before corrections are made, you can usually determine approximately the required degree of past pointing.

You should also notice in Figure 10.8 that the dose gradient directly above the hot region is very great; i.e., the dose falls off very rapidly to an uneffective value. If you past point and don't take this gradient into account, you run the risk of completely missing a portion of the target volume.

Past pointing is required with more than two fields if they are all directed from the same hemisphere. While this is rarely, if ever, done with individual fixed fields, it occurs in arc therapy, to be discussed later. When the arc used is less than 360°, some past pointing is necessary.

F.
Two-Field Isodose Summations in SSD Planning

There are, generally speaking, only two cases - opposing and non-opposing fields. Since we just looked at the case of non-opposing fields and considered the techniques of isodose

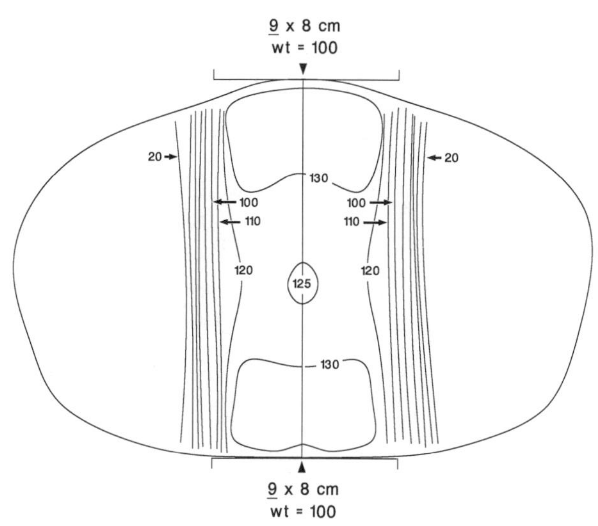

Figure 10.10. Isodose summation of an opposing equally weighted pair.

summation, we will now consider isodose summation in the case of opposing pairs.

There are again two possible types of fields - equally weighted and unequally weighted. Figure 10.11 is a typical example of an isodose summation for an opposing equally weighted pair. As we noted earlier, the departure from homogeneity is not great in the full primary region. This distribution tends to be less homogenous in the direction parallel to the central rays if the fields are small, the patient is thick, the radiation is "soft," or the SSD is short. Figure 10.11 illustrates a 2:1 weighting.

Figure 10.12 shows the effect of parallel fields directed through non-parallel surfaces. This situation will be encountered frequently in two locations; in treatment of the anterior of the neck region, such as the larynx, and the tangential chest wall or breast. Note the shift away from homogeneity, with the high dose occurring in the thinner portion of the anatomy.

Figure 10.11. Isodose summation of an opposing unequally weighted pair.

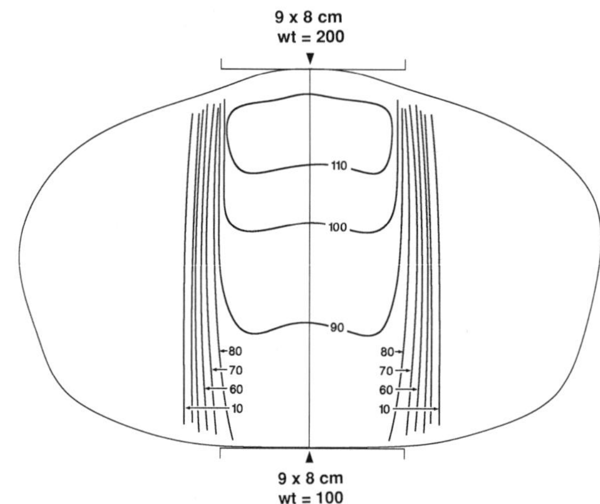

Figure 10.12. Isodose distributions of an opposing equally weighted pair incidence on non-parallel surface.

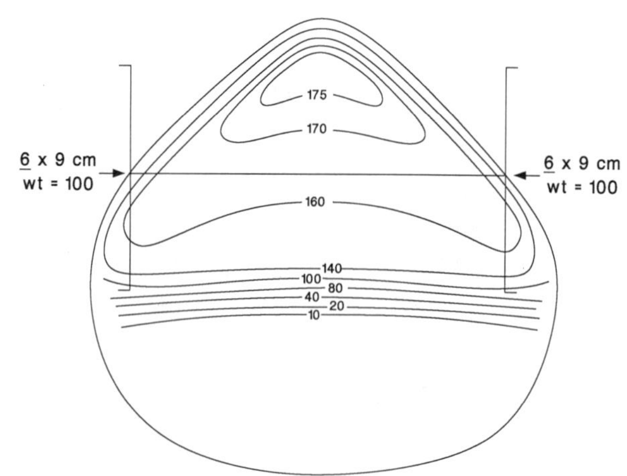

G.
Multiple Opposing Pairs in SSD Planning

The basic patterns for opposing pairs can be combined into four field and six field techniques in various ways. Four fields consisting of two opposing pairs are used in what is frequently called the **box technique.** Figure 10.13 shows the box technique when all four fields are equally weighted. Figure 10.14 shows the summation when one pair is equally weighted but has a different weight than that of the other pair.

Note in each case that the highest dose encountered is at the target volume, and that it is significantly higher than at any point of d_{max}. This is the advantage of this technique over a single opposing pair. The obvious disadvantage is that more tissue is irradiated (integral dose is higher).

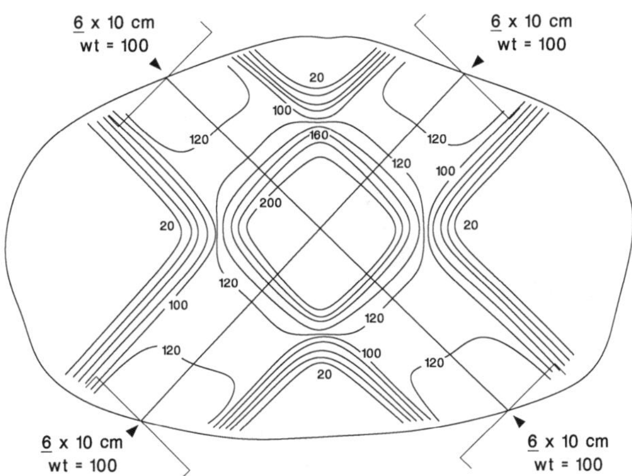

Figure 10.13. Four fields of two opposing, equally weighted pairs.

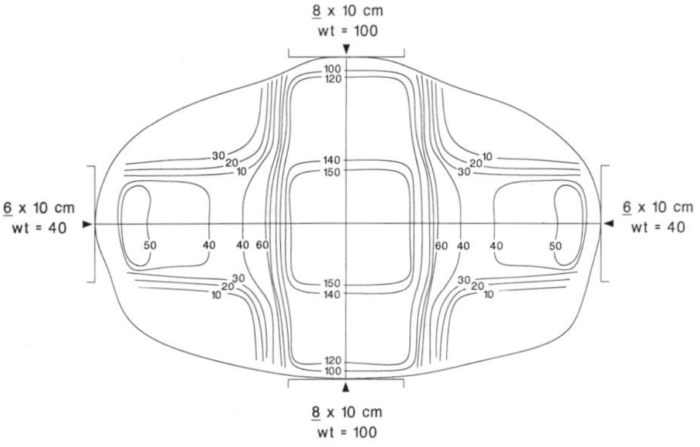

Figure 10.14. Four fields of two opposing pairs, in which one pair has different weighting than the other pair.

H.
Three Field Technique in SSD Planning

Figure 10.15 shows an isodose summation for a typical 3-field technique. These may be used as an anterior and two oblique posterior, or vice versa. Sometimes the technique can involve equally weighted fields, but often the oblique pair is weighted somewhat less than the third field (as in the case of Figure 10.15).

This technique is often used to treat the esophagus or bladder region. An alternative approach is arc therapy.

Figure 10.15. Isodose distribution of 3-field technique. Posterior oblique fields are weighted differently than the anterior field.

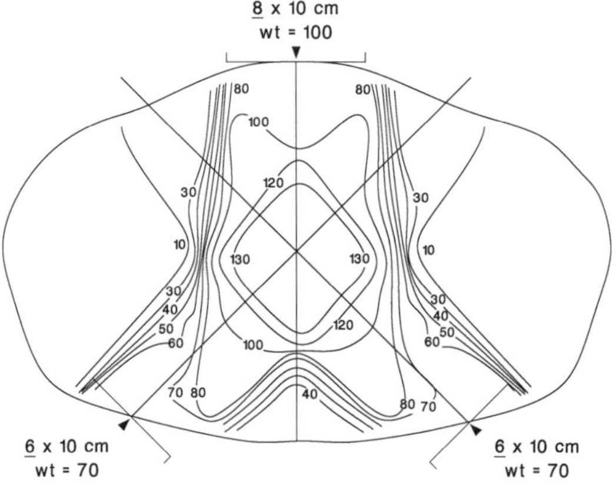

I.
Isodose Curves for SAD Planning

Thus far, all of the summations presented have been for SSD plans. Figure 10.16 shows a single field isodose map which could be used for SAD planning.

Observe the differences between isodose curves and the curves used for SSD planning: while the shapes of the individual isodose curves are similar to those used for SSD planning, the values assigned to them are normalized at 10 cm depth (the isocenter in this case), rather than at d_{max}. The field size is specified at 10 cm depth (the isocenter) and obviously there are lines whose values are greater than 100%.

A similar set of curves may be normalized at 5 cm or 15 cm depth. This does not mean that you can only use these curves if the axis (isocenter) lies at a depth of 5, 10, or 15 cm. If, for example, the axis in a particular case is at a depth of 8 cm, you would find an isodose map for that field size which is normalized near the depth in question (in this case, 10 cm) and proceed as if there were no difference between the depth in question and the normalization depth of the isodose map. You will find it most convenient to pick a distribution with a normalization depth just greater than the axis depth in the particular treatment you are planning.

The error involved in the above assumption is actually not as great as the error in assuming a semi-infinite patient.

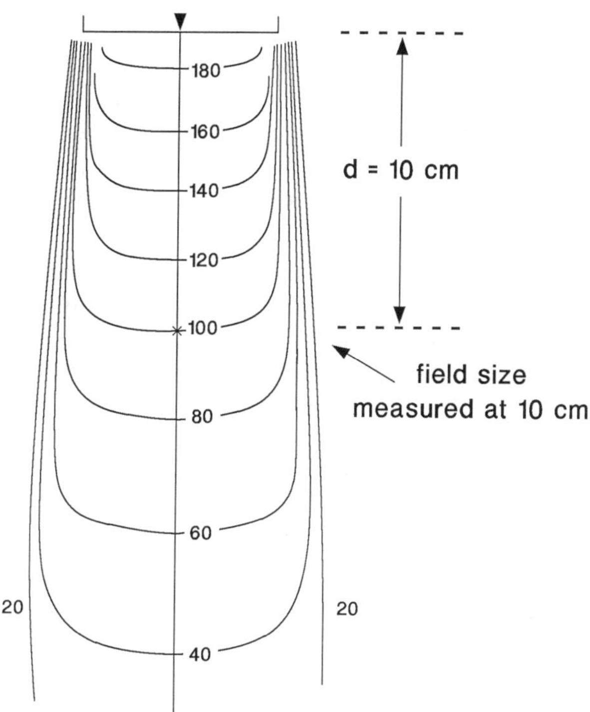

Figure 10.16.
Isodose pattern for
SAD planning.

J.
Isodose Summation using SAD Type Isodose Curves

The methods discussed for compensating for skin curvature by shifting isodose lines, for adjusting the values of the curves for different field weights, and for actual isodose summation are exactly the same as for SSD isodose planning. The only differences are that the individual field isodose patterns are positioned by aligning their normalization points at the axis chosen for the plan and that the summed value of the isodose curves at the axis (isocenter) will always equal the sum of the weights of all fields used.

Interpretation of the values of the summed lines and the use of TMR's or TAR's to calculate treatment duration were discussed in Chapter 11.

K.
Isodose Summation by Computer

Isodose summation by hand is a lengthy procedure, as you now know. You must choose entry points, field sizes, angles, etc., before beginning, and you must determine these variables using a combination of intuition, clinical experience, and luck. Thus if the plan does not quite accomplish what you set out to accomplish, but could be improved by shifting one or more of the above parameters, you will have a tendency to accept the plan as is anyway, rather than repeat the entire process. This is one disadvantage of isodose summation by hand.

Modern computer techniques allow you to plan a relatively complicated treatment, complete with isodose summation, in about one half hour. An advantage of computer techniques is that if you don't like the plan, you can quickly alter any or all of the parameters in a matter of minutes. Obviously, both you and the patient benefit.

Why should you learn to do isodose summation by hand if the computer can do it faster (and possibly, but not necessarily, more accurately)? There are a number of excellent reasons, including the obvious fact that you may not have access to a computer.

Computers break down and the more complex the computer, the greater the likelihood of malfunction. During this "down time," you will probably not wish to suspend all treatment planning.

The individual steps used in hand summations of isodose curves may appear on board examinations, so it is wise to become familiar with them.

A computer is an underling. The mark of a good boss is to know the jobs of his underlings well enough to perform them him or herself. This enables the boss to better assess the work of the underling.

If you are experienced in doing summations by hand, you will find computer planning easier. You cannot show the patient to the computer and say, "Computer, give me a plan to cure this patient!" Instead, you must still decide how many fields to use, how to weight and orient them, etc. With personal experience behind you, you will find yourself creating satisfactory plans by computer on the first attempt.

References

1. Johns, H.E. & Cunningham, J.R. *The Physics of Radiology*, 4th Edition, Charles C. Thomas, 1983, pp. 358-388.
2. Hendee, W.R. *Radiation Therapy Physics*, 2nd Edition, Year Book Medical Publishers, 1981, pp. 117-120.
3. Khan, F.M. *The Physics of Radiation Therapy*, Williams & Wilkins, 1984, pp. 249-254.
4. International Commission on Radiation Units and Measurements, Report 24, *Determination of Absorbed Dose in a Patient Irradiated by Beams of X or Gamma Rays in Radiotherapy Procedures*, Washington, D.C., United States National Bureau of Standards, 1976, pp. 19-21.
5. Ibid., p. 21.
6. Giessen, I. "A Method of Calculating the Isodose Shift in Correcting for Oblique Incidence in Radiotherapy," *British Journal of Radiology*, 46:978-982, 1973.

Wedge Filters

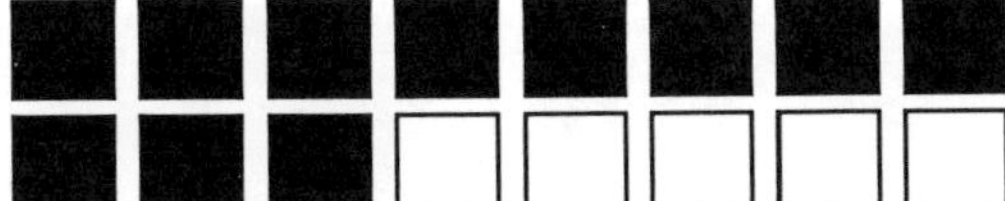

11

In Chapter 10 we looked at the case of two non-opposing fields and found that the resulting dose summation pattern had a great many faults. Nevertheless, there are many occasions when the only sensible treatment involves two obliquely directed fields. Head and neck problems, for example, involve critical constraints on the treatment plan, such as the eyes, the tangential surfaces of the lips, the ears and the upper spinal cord, even though the target volume involved occupies a significant fraction of the total volume of the anatomy. Opposing field, despite their simplicity and usual freedom from "hot" and "cold" spots, are often avoided because of these constraints.

Wedge filters often solve problems associated with using opposing fields.[1-8] They are often merely called "wedges;" the use of the term "filter" is ill advised. A filter is a device for modifying the quality or hardness of a beam, but the wedge filter is designed to modify the distribution of a beam.

A.
Wedge Angle

A wedge filter is a wedge shaped attenuator; it is placed at the end of the collimator so that electrons ejected from the wedge will not contaminate the photon beam. In addition, this prevents the dose buildup effect on the patient's surface. The minimum collimator to skin distance varies approximately as much as 15-25 cm for photon energies ranging from cobalt-60 to 24 MV. More radiation penetrates the thin end of the wedge than the thick end.

The wedge, in cross section, looks like Figure 11.1 (a) or (b).

Figure 11.1 (a) and (b). Wedge cross-sections.

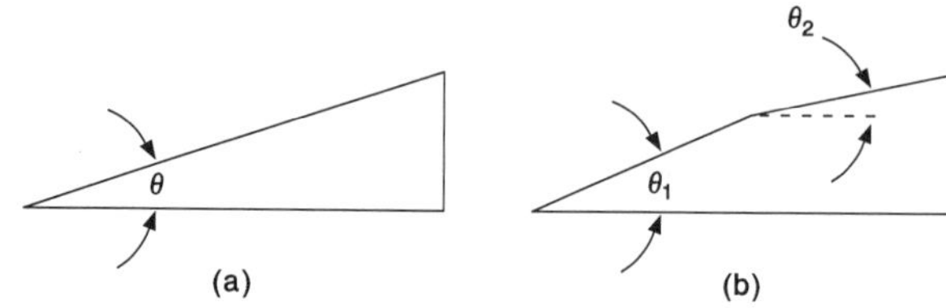

The angle in Figure 11.1 depends not only on the intended purpose of the wedge, but also on the wedge material (usually lead, but wedges of brass, steel, aluminum, and even hardwood have been used).

The term **wedge angle** (usually some multiple of 15°) does not refer to the angle θ as pictured in Figure 11.1. In fact, the wedge angle is not any angle on the wedge at all, but refers to the effect on the isodose curves.[9] The wedge angle is defined as the angle of tilt of an isodose curve (the angle between the isodose curve and a line perpendicular to the central ray) along the central ray of a beam and at a specified depth, usually recommended to be 10 cm.[10]

B.
Conditions for Homogeneity

There is a useful mental device for determining how homogeneity can be achieved. At any point on an isodose curve, we can construct a tangent line. Then from the point we can construct a line perpendicular to the tangent line and assign to it a direction (indicated by an arrowhead) and a magnitude. For magnitude, we shall choose the rate at which dose is changing along the direction of the arrow. For the direction, we can only choose between increasing or decreasing dose. Figure 11.2 illustrates these ideas.

We will call this arrow the **gradient** of the field at that point (i.e., the point at which the tangent line touches the isodose curve).

Note that the gradient in the penumbra region of the field in Figure 11.2 is drawn larger than the gradients in the full primary portion of the field. Remember that the magnitude we assigned to the gradient relates to the rate of change of dose and not to the actual amount of dose. The rate of change of dose in the penumbra is very great.

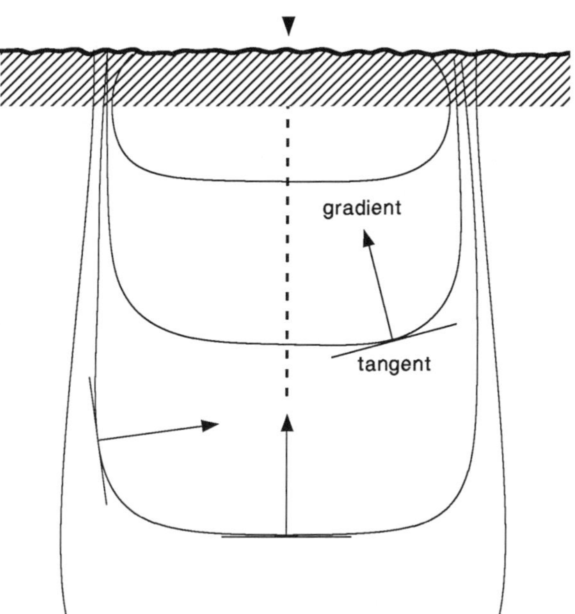

We will use the concept of gradient to better understand the conditions for homogeneity when more than one field is involved in the treatment plan. We will further extend our concept by multiplying the gradients by the relative weight of the field, calling the result the **weighted gradient.**

The weighted gradient will be larger if either the dose is high or the rate of change is great (or both).

We have thus far encountered a number of cases in which a reasonably good dose homogeneity was accomplished using multiple fields, i.e., with equally weighted opposing fields, with various combinations of pairs of equally weighted opposing fields (Figures 10.12, 10.13), and with the three field technique of Figure 10.14. In each case, homogeneity was good where all fields contributed to the dose and not good otherwise.

Figure 11.3 (a), (b), (c) and (d) is a representation of the gradients of the isodose summations of Figures 10.12, 10.13 and 10.14, as well as the case of opposing fields.

Note that in each case, where all fields combine, the weighted gradients cancel each other (like a number of equally strong oxen pulling in different directions), and that these are the regions where the dose homogeneity is greatest.

If the weighted gradients of two or more fields can be made to cancel, homogeneity will occur.

*11.3 (a) weighted
gradient represen-
tation of opposing
equally wieghted
beams.
(b) weighted gra-
dients for the box
technique of Figure
10.12.*

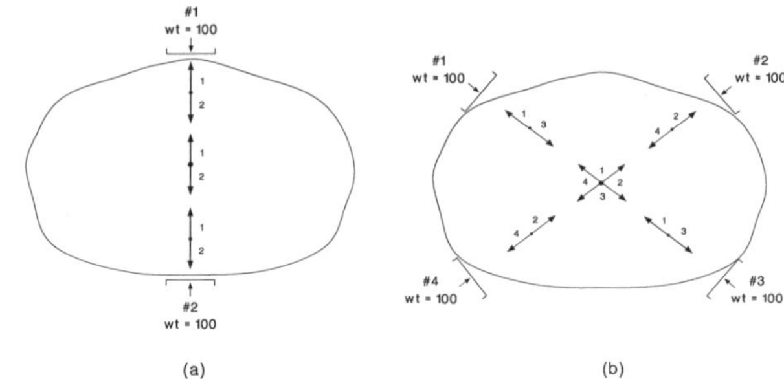

(a)   (b)

*(c) weighted
gradients for the
box technique of
Figure 10.13.
(d) weighted
gradients for the
3-field technique of
Figure 10.14.*

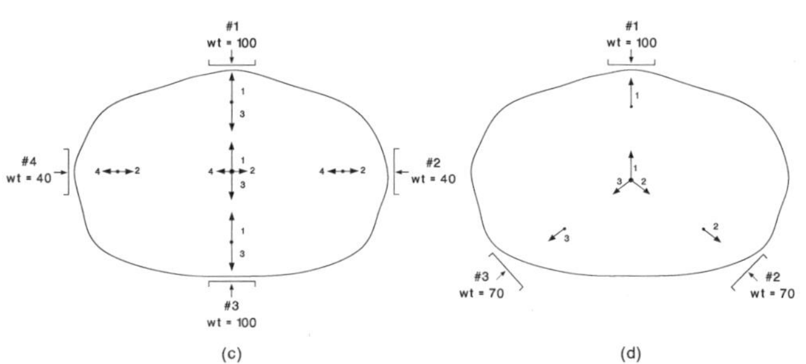

(c)   (d)

Now let us look at the three cases we encountered in which homogeneity did not occur: the non-parallel fields of Figure 10.6; the opposing but unequally weighted fields of Figure 10.10; and the opposing pair directed through non-parallel surfaces of Figure 10.11.

*Figure 11.4.
(a) Weighted
gradients in the
case of Figure 10.6.
(b) Weighted
gradients in the
case of Figure
10.10.
(c) Weighted
gradients in the
case of Figure
10.11.*

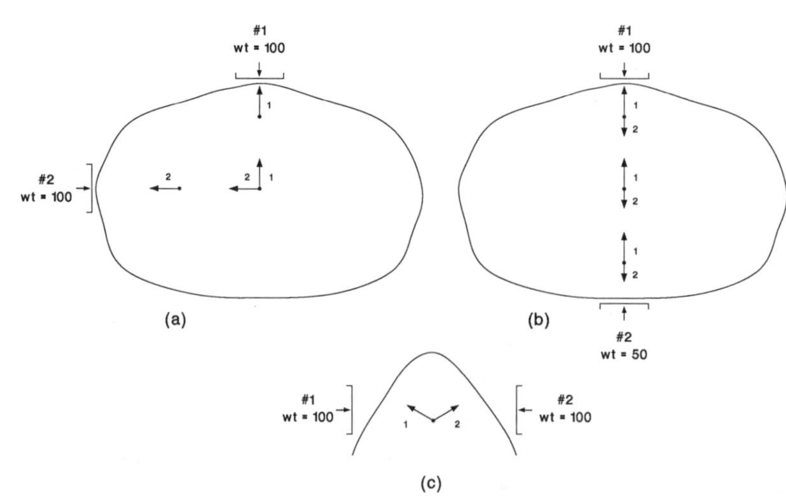

(a)   (b)

(c)

In Figure 11.4 (a), the gradients do not cancel because they do not "pull" in opposite directions. In Figure 11.4 (b) they do not cancel because the gradient of field 1 "outpulls" that of field 2; and in Figure 11.4 (c), they are not pulling in strictly opposite positions because the sloping skin surface has shifted the isodose curves, and thus shifted the gradients.

Homogeneity can be accomplished by controlling either field weights, gradient directions, or both. No choice of weights will accomplish homogeneity in Figure 11.4 (a) or (c); homogeneity requires a change in the directions of the gradients, as pictured in Figure 11.5.

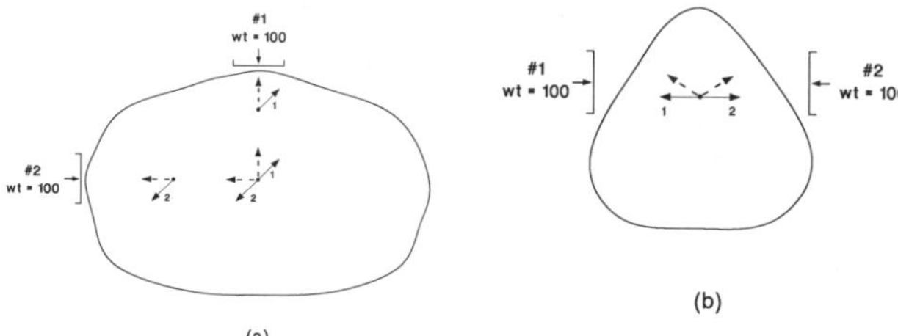

Figure 11.5. Homogeneity accomplished by shifting the weighted gradients through an angle of about (a) 45°; and (b) 30°.

The direction of the weight gradient is perpendicular to the tangent of the isodose curve at that point. In order to shift the direction of the gradient by 45°, you would have to tilt the isodose curves by this angle. Thus an isodose distribution for fields used to accomplish homogeneity in the case of an obliquely directed pair of fields like those in Fig. 11.5 (a) would look like Fig. 11.6:

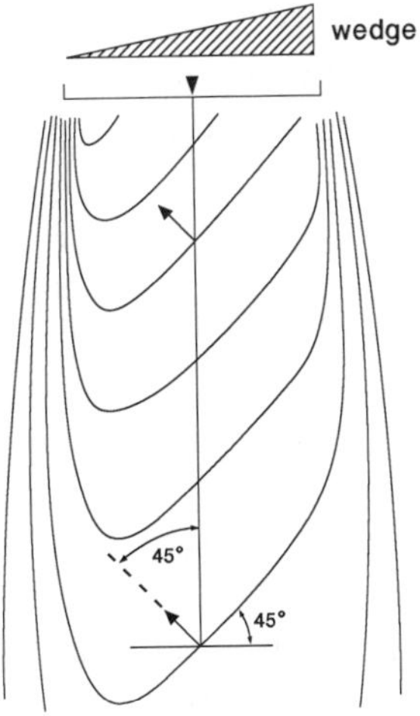

Figure 11.6. Use of a wedge filter to shift the field gradient.

This is accomplished by means of a wedge filter. The wedge angle is the angle through which the gradient is shifted in the central part of the field; for example, 45° in Figure 11.6.

Thus, using wedge filters, you can achieve homogeneity (or nearly so) in cases such as those pictured in Figures 10.6 and 10.11, as well as in other situations.

C.
Hinge Angle

Wedge filters are normally used in pairs, although sometimes these pairs are used in conjunction with other fields. When homogeneity is required using just two weighted fields, only one hinge angle will accomplish the homogeneity, given a wedge angle.

The hinge angle is the angle between the central rays of two fields (for example, 90° in Figure 10.6). A simple relationship exists between hinge angle and wedge angle, which is strictly valid only when the beams of radiation are directed perpendicular to the skin [i.e., it would be erroneous for a case such as pictured in Figure 11.5(b)]. This relationship is:

$$hinge\ angle\ =\ 180°\text{-}\ 2\ (wedge\ angle)$$

Wedge Angle	Hinge Angle
15°	180° - 2 (15°) = 180° - 30° = 150°
30°	180° - 2 (30°) = 180° - 60° = 120°
45°	180° - 2 (45°) = 180° - 90° = 90°
60°	180° - 2 (60°) = 180° - 120° = 60°

In reality, sloping skin surfaces change these ideal angles somewhat. For example, you might find that better homogeneity is often accomplished using a hinge angle of 95° to 100° with 45° wedges.

D.
Wedge Factor

In using wedge filters, there is a trade-off in obtaining a good distribution because of the lengthy procedures needed to obtain the distribution. By introducing lead in front of the collimator, you reduce the dose rate and lengthen the treatment time. The fraction of the beam which survives through the wedge at central ray is called the **wedge factor,** or **wedge attenuation factor.** It is defined as the ratio of output with and without the wedge at the depth of maximum dose along the central ray in a maxiphantom.

There are two distinct ways to orient a wedge filter in a beam. The simplest is to fix the wedge support so that the wedge always slides into the same position, as in Figure 11.7. This means that the same portion of the wedge is always in the path of the central ray, regardless of the field size. Hence the wedge factor will change only very slightly due to field size.

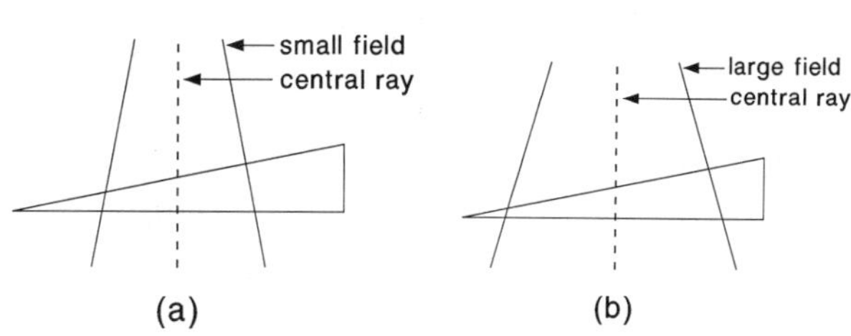

Figure 11.7. Wedge filter position in a beam, fixed wedge position.

The problem with this wedge orientation is that for a small field, a large portion of the material of the wedge is not acting as a wedge, but as an overall beam intensity reducer. (This is true for any field size, but more so for small fields).

Figure 11.8

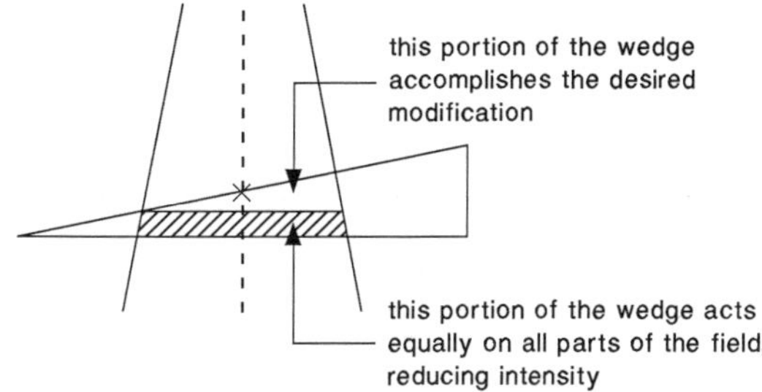

This second method uses the minimum amount of lead necessary to edge the field and thus maximizes the dose rate, but it also calls for a significantly more complicated wedge alignment procedure, meaning that the wedge factor will vary widely as a function of field size. Thus it is easier to make a serious mistake.

Figure 11.9 (a) and (b). Wedge shifts laterally to keep thin end at field's edge.

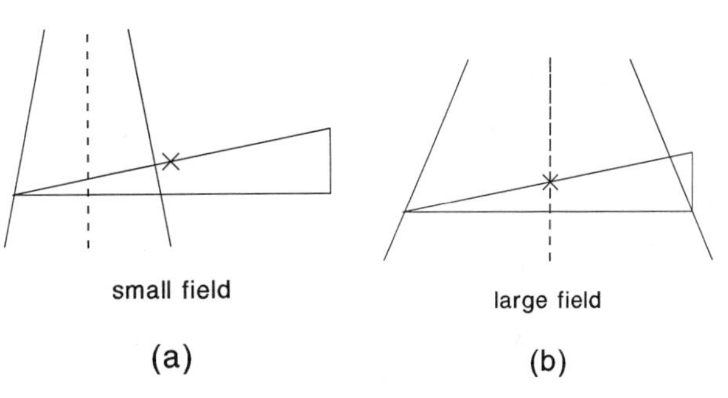

Since dose rate is not a problem with modern linear accelerators, the first method is normally used.

There are also a variety of ways of normalizing the isodose distribution for a wedged field. At least four ways are in common use - two for SAD technique and two for SSD technique. When the values are normalized at d_{max} for SSD techniques, then two interpretations of the meaning of the percentage values assigned to the isodose lines can be made. For example, the dose on the 60% line may be 60% of the dose at d_{max} with the wedge in place, or 60% of the dose for an open field of the same size (i.e., at d_{max} without the wedge). Figure 11.10 shows these two presentations for the same field.

Figure 11.10

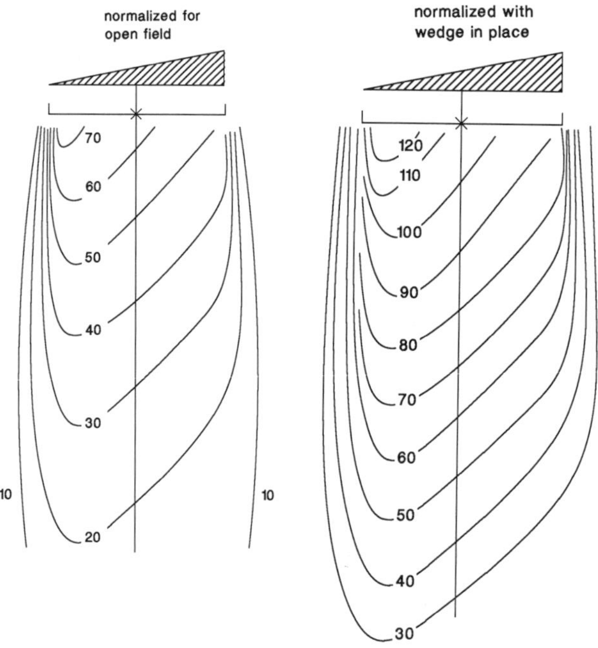

The wedge factor is the ratio of the values of the assigned dose percentage in the two representations of Figure 11.10. That is, if you choose any point in the field of the first representation and multiply the wedge factor by the values assigned to the isodose curve at that point, you will achieve the assigned value of the isodose curve at that point in the second representation. In particular, since the point on the central ray at d_{max} is automatically assigned a value of 100%, then the value of this point in the second representation is equal to the wedge factor, expressed as a percentage.

If you have done an isodose summation using isodose distributions of the first type (normalized with the wedge in place), then the calculation for treatment duration must contain the wedge factor.

$$T = \frac{D_p \cdot weight}{CAL \cdot I_p \cdot (W \cdot F)}$$

where "weight" is the weight expressed as a fraction (its decimal value), w is the wedge factor and I_p is the decimal value of the isodose line which is chosen for the prescription dose.

On the other hand, if you have used isodose distributions of the second kind (normalized at d_{max} with no wedge), then the wedge factor is already present in the isodose values, and should not appear in the calculation.

$$T = \frac{D_p \cdot weight}{CAL \cdot I_p}$$

In the case of SAD planning, isodose values may also be normalized at an isocenter depth with or without the wedge factor. As in open field planning, the TMR (or TAR) must appear in the calculation of treatment duration. In the equations below, D_{iso} is the dose required at isocenter to achieve the prescription dose within the chosen isodose line, and I_{iso} is the sum of all weights (see Chapter 9):

$$T = \frac{D_{iso} \cdot weight}{TMR \cdot w \cdot I_{iso} \cdot CAL}$$

for a distribution normalized at isocenter with wedge in place (i.e., isodose line at isocenter on central ray has value 100), or:

$$T = \frac{D_{iso} \cdot weight}{TMR \cdot I_{iso} \cdot CAL}$$

for a distribution normalized at axis to open field value (i.e., isodose line at axis on central ray has value equal to wedge factor).

Notice in the above that the ratio D_{iso} / I_{iso} appears. Since $D_{iso} = D_p (I_{iso} / I_p)$, this simplifies to $D_p = I_p$; therefore, you need not truly calculate the dose at the isocenter. Treatment duration may be calculated solely on the basis of prescription dose at the prescription isodose line. In Chapter 9, it was recommended that you first find the dose at the isocenter and use the TMR to calculate treatment duration. This procedure was recommended so that you could see how each field contributed to the treatment. The only point at which this can readily be seen is at the isocenter, where all TMR's are referred. In this case, the result will be the same if you calculate treatment duration using D_p and I_p, without ever referring to the isocenter dose, using the equation below. However, it is still recommended that you calculate the dose at the isocenter, since this is always a critical point in the treatment plan. You may then calculate treatment duration using the steps outlined in Chapter 9. The following general equation is the shortest route in calculating dose at the isocenter, and may be used as a check.

In general, for any field using SAD planning:

$$T = \frac{D_{pc} \cdot weight}{TMR \cdot w \cdot CAL \cdot I_p \cdot N_c}$$

where D_{pc} is the prescription dose per cycle time; N_c is the number of times this field is used per cycle; I_p is the isodose value at the prescription point or at the boundary of the target volume selected for prescription dose; TMR may be TAR or TPR, depending on the nature of CAL. The w is the wedge factor. It will equal 1.0 if (a) no wedge is used, or (b) the isodose distribution used was normalized to an open field value, which means the isodose line at axis has a value equal to the wedge factor.

Weight is expressed in the same terms as I_p. For example, if I_p is a decimal value such as 1.6, then weight will be a decimal value such as 0.5; or if Ip = 160, then weight will be 50. Note that weight expresses the relative dose at the normalization point, rather than the relative treatment duration.

A corresponding general equation for SSD planning is:

$$T = \frac{D_{pc} \cdot weight}{w \cdot CAL \cdot I_p \cdot N_c}$$

where I_p is interpreted as before, but can be equal to ddf_p for simple dosimetry with single or equally weighted fields. $w = 1.0$ if (a) no wedge is used, or (b) the value of the isodose line on the central ray at d_{max} is equal to the wedge factor (field is normalized to open field value).

E.
Some Wedge Filter Isodose Summations

First we should see how wedge filters can be used to improve the treatment plan represented in Figure 10.6 and discussed in the last section. Figure 11.11 shows the isodose summations using unwedged fields and the obvious improvements in homogeneity when 45° wedged fields are used.

Observe in Figure 11.11 that the thick portions of the wedge

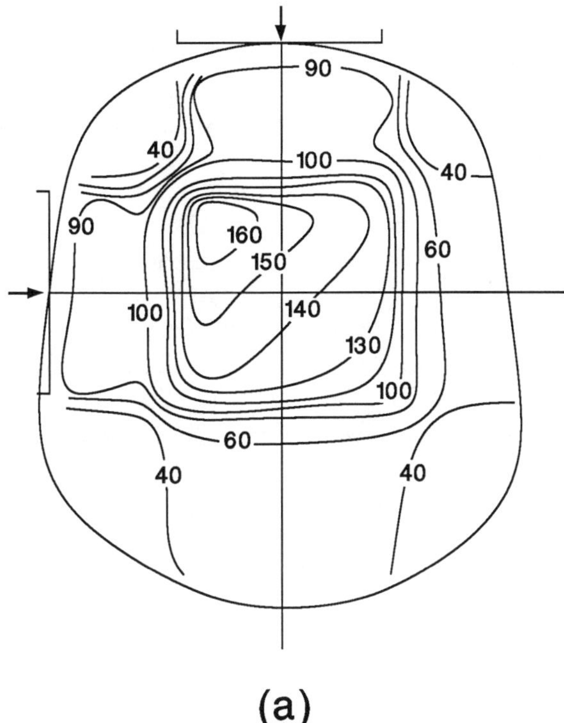

(a)

Figure 11 (a). Isodose summation of two 6 x 6 cm open fields at right angles (Clinac-4).

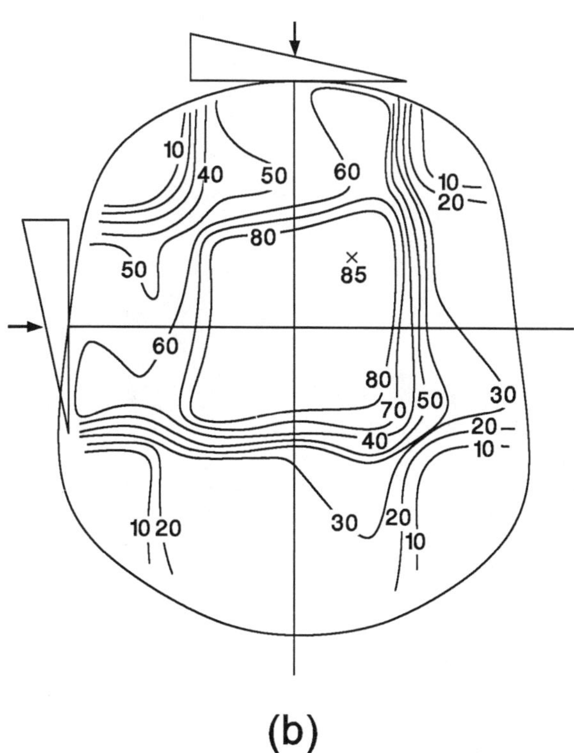

(b)

Figure 11 (b). Same situation using 45° wedge filters.

are oriented toward each other. Remember from our previous discussion of gradients that the gradient for a wedged field is always tilted away from the vertical toward the thin edge of the wedge, as in Figure 11.12 (a). Figures 11.12 (b), and (c) and (d) indicate what happens when the wedges are oriented in various ways with respect to one another. In (b), homogeneity will occur, indicated by the cancelling of gradients. In (c), the effect of the wedges cancels out, and an isodose summation would be very similar to that using unwedged fields. In (d), there is a great departure from homogeneity. You should now see that you must be very careful with the alignment of wedges.

Figures 11.13 (a) and (b) show isodose summations for typical treatment plans using 60° and 30° wedges. Obviously, the shape of the target volume (and the physical constraints such as the presence of eyes, etc.) will dictate the choice of wedge angle.

Figure 11.12. (a) Gradient always tilts off central ray toward thin edge of wedge.
(b) Wedges aligned correctly; gradients cancel.

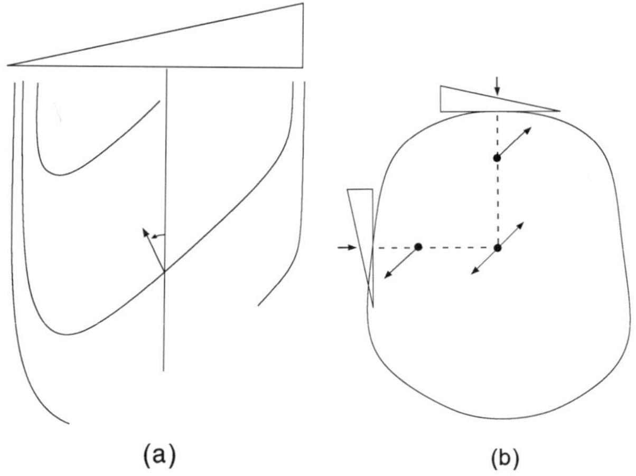

(a)   (b)

(c) One wedge incorrectly aligned; amount of inhomogeneity equivalent to open field plan.
(d) Both wedges incorrectly aligned; very great inhomogeneity.

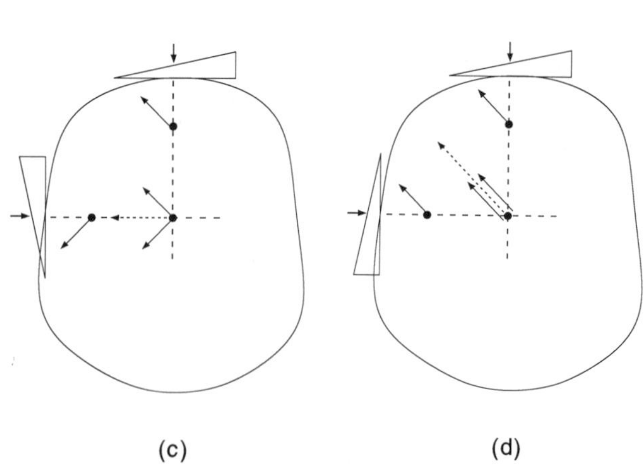

(c)   (d)

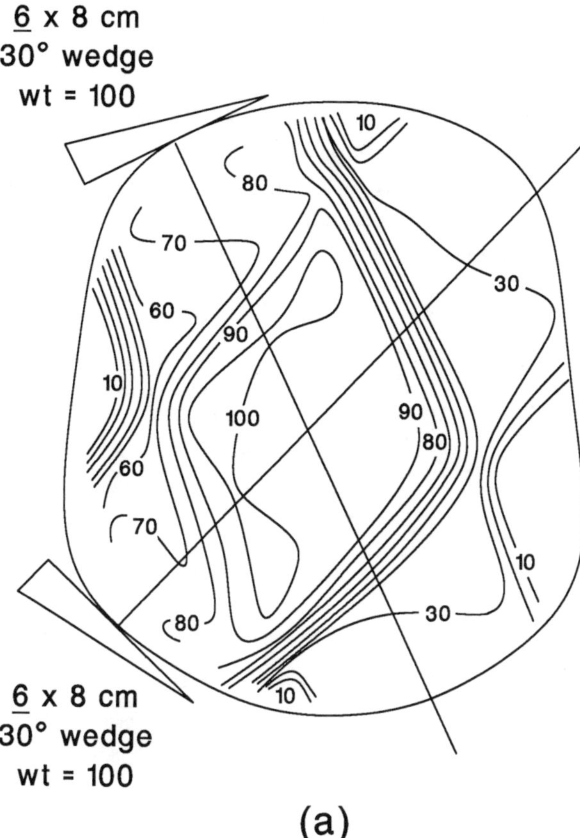

Figure 11.13. (a) Treatment plan using 30° wedge.

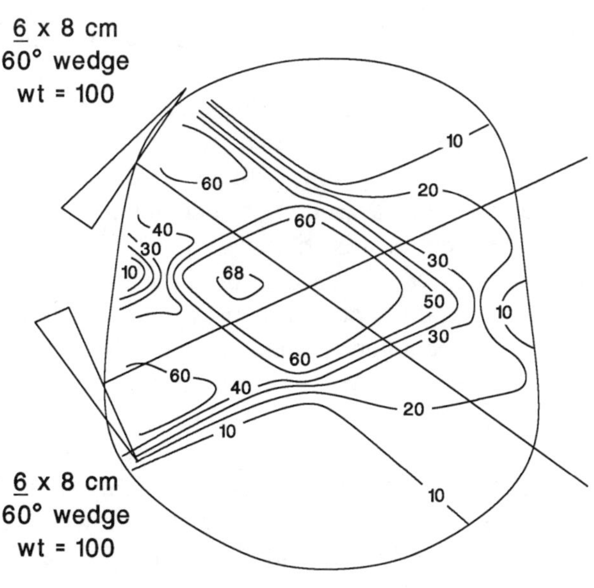

(b) Treatment plan using 60° wedge.

Figure 11.14 shows what happens when you use a wedge pair with a hinge angle other than that required by the hinge versus wedge angle equation (see section C). Note the departure from homogeneity, which can be seen when a gradient representation of the plan is drawn.

Figure 11.14

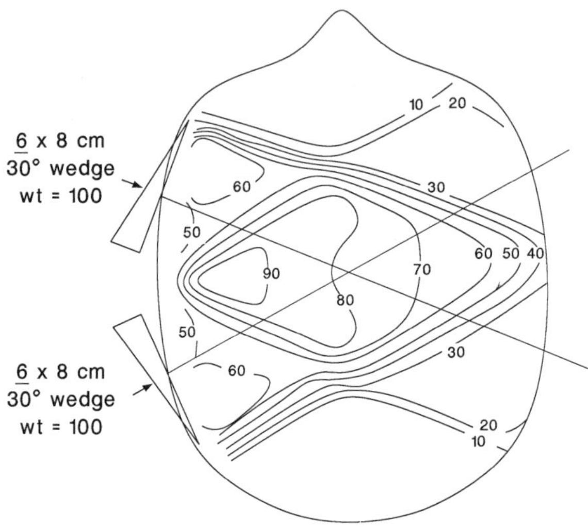

F.
Wedge Plans Using Opposing Wedges

There are a few occasions when you intentionally use wedged fields at angles greatly different from calculated hinge angles. According to the hinge angle formula, for example, if the hinge angle is 180°, the wedge angle should be zero, and thus the field is not wedged. Recall, however, that the optimum hinge angle changes for a beam entering skin with a sloped contour. In such cases, the tissue itself has a wedging effect and a wedge filter can be used to compensate for this "tissue-wedge."

Opposing wedges can be used in the case in Chapter 10, for example, where a parallel opposed pair of fields entered the non-parallel surfaces of the anterior neck. This was one of our examples of non-homogeneity. We will now use 30° wedges to improve the homogeneity (see Figure 11.15).

Another example of the use of parallel opposed wedges occurs in the following common problem. In Figure 11.16, the cross section of a head contains a target volume which has certain constraints. It has been decided that the right eye will be sacrificed, since it has diseased tissue. You would hope, however, to spare the left eye, not only from loss of function, but also from later cataract formation, which takes only approximately 4 Gy over a normally scheduled time (5 weeks). In addition, it is necessary to treat the tissues far anterior, in the bridge of the nose between the eyes, and to treat all tissues on the right side of the head to a posterior depth of 8 cm. Within this volume, we must treat all tissue to a dose of 60 Gy ± 10%. You are encouraged to try your hand at treatment plans to accomplish this goal other than those below.

Figure 11.15

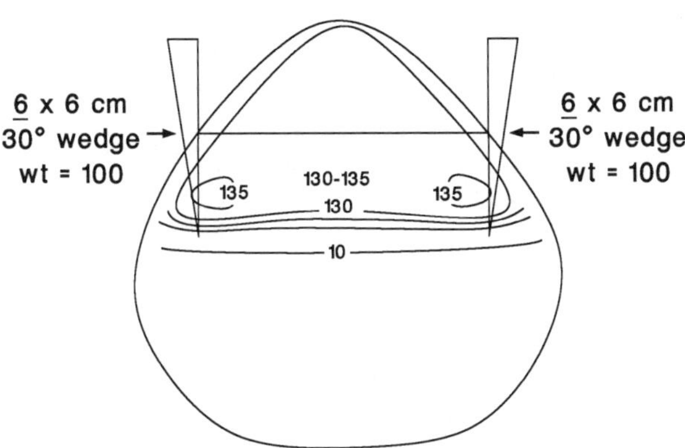

*Figure 11.16.
Cross section of a
head.*

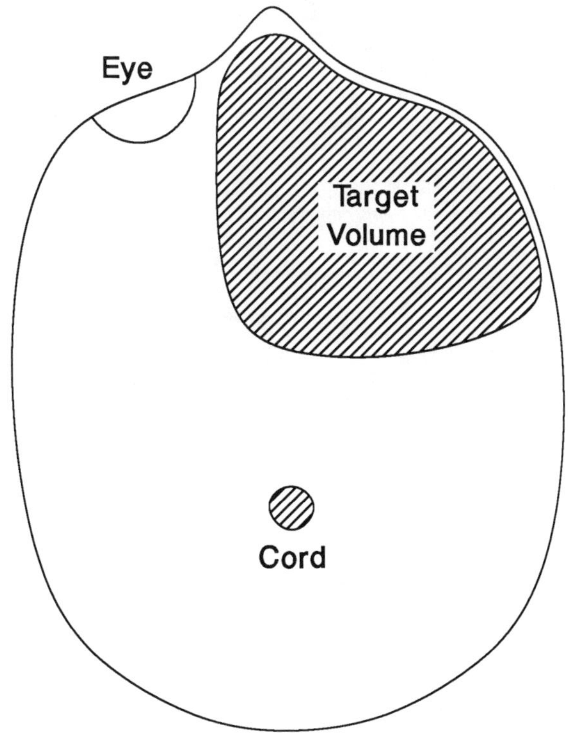

In Figure 11.17 consider two obvious plans for treating the patient, ignoring the constraints.

Figure 11.17. (a) Pair of parallel opposed beams.

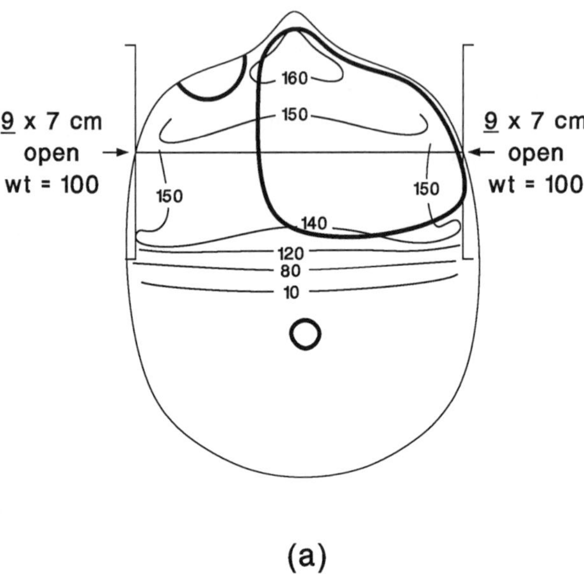

(a)

(b) Wedge pair of beams with hinge angle of 90°.

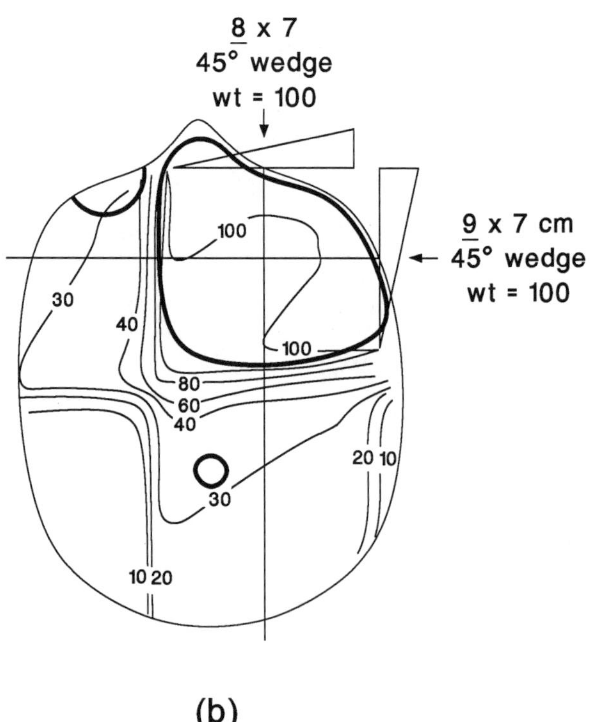

(b)

Obviously these plans treat the diseased tissue to the specified tolerance, but sacrifice both eyes, and are therefore not acceptable.

If the lateral field of Figure 11.17 (b) could be angled back somewhat, dose to the lens of the left eye would be reduced. This would require a smaller hinge angle than 90°, and now 60°, instead of 45°, wedges (see Figure 11.18).

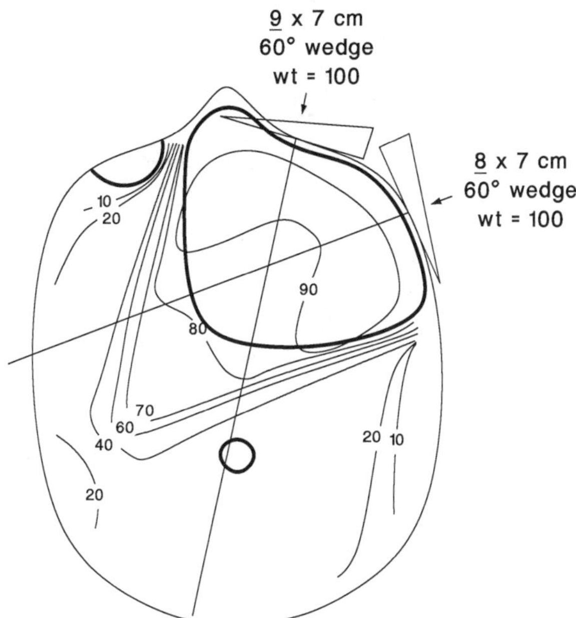

Figure 11.18. Wedge pair of beams with hinge angle smaller than 90°.

This plan is marginally acceptable, but has two major faults. First, the left eye is only partially spared. In order to insure that the anterior aspects of the target volume are treated, it is necessary to cut the margin at the left orbit rather close. Daily inconsistency in the actual set-up of the patient in the treatment room would create a risk of cataract formation. Secondly, a high dose area occurs across midline on the posterior left side. You would like to lessen the dose there, if possible.

Figure 11.19 shows the simplest approach for this treatment, a single anterior field.

This approach obviously spares the good eye, but the variation in dose is greater than ± 10% throughout the target volume. If there were some way to "boost" the dose in the posterior portion of the target volume, we would have an acceptable plan. This could be done with a pair of opposing open fields used laterally with their anterior borders beginning behind the eye; but such a pair would, by themselves, have a zero gradient (homogeneity). The anterior field they are supposed to boost has a

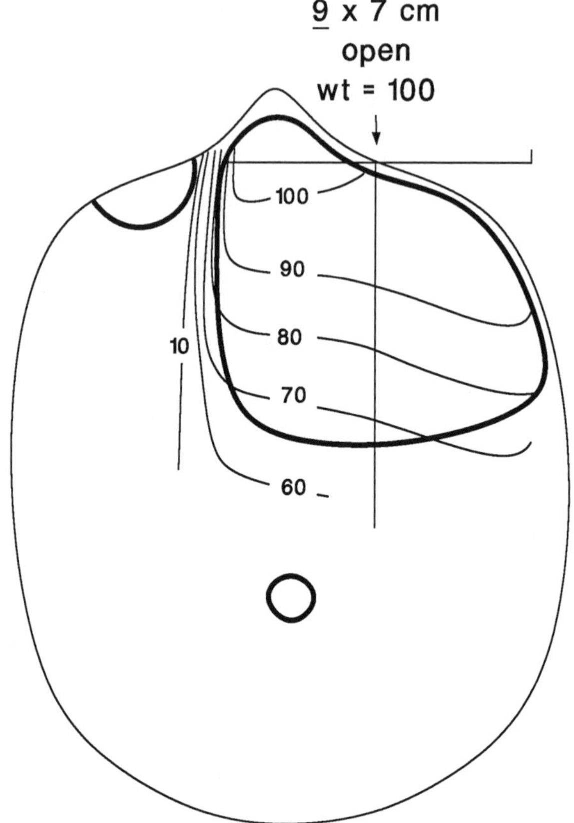

gradient, pictured in Figure 11.19, directed forward and tilted slightly toward the right due to skin curvature. An opposing pair of lateral wedges would direct the gradient posteriorly (if they are applied with the thick ends forward).

You can match the magnitude of the anterior field gradient by adjusting the combined weights of the wedged pair. You can then "tilt" the gradient of the wedged pair by adjusting the relative weights of the two wedges. By tinkering with these parameters, you can achieve a gradient for the wedged pair which will directly oppose and cancel the gradient of the anterior field, thus achieving homogeneity in the volume treated by all three fields. The remaining inhomogeneity will be confined to the anterior field, and this may easily be kept within the ± 10% tolerance.

Figure 11.20 illustrates the effect of changes in these parameters on the pair of opposing wedged fields.

In Figure 11.21 you will see the combination of all three fields for a successful treatment plan.

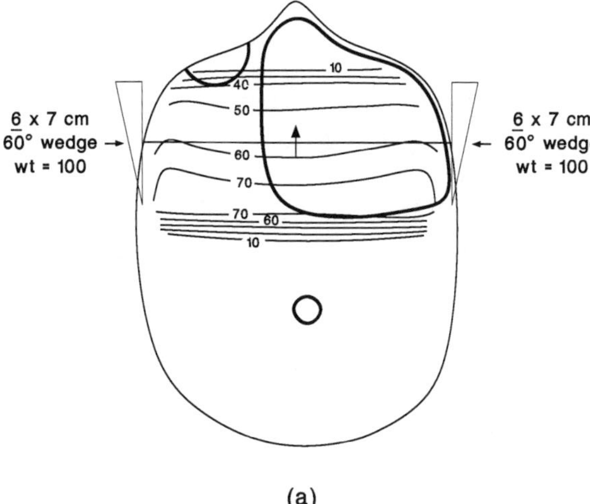

(a)

*Figure 11.20. (a)
An opposing pair of
lateral wedges with
60° wedge.*

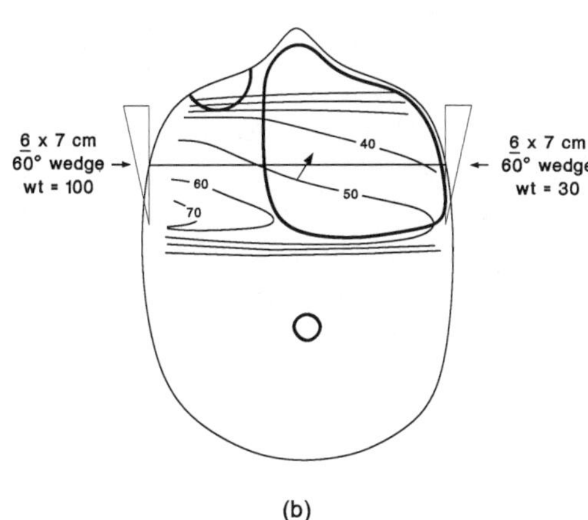

(b)

*(b) An opposing
pair of lateral
wedges with a 60°
and 30° wedge,
respectively.*

Figure 11.21

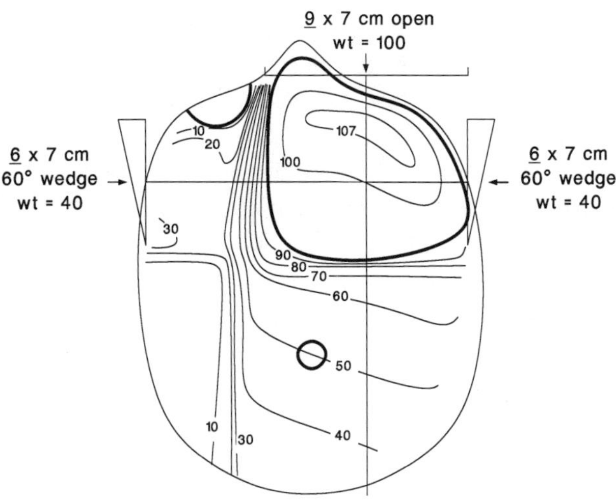

G.
Using Wedged and Open Fields in Combination to Simulate Lesser Wedge Angles

Wedge filters normally have wedge angles of 30°, 45°, and/or 60° (and sometimes 15°). These are sufficient to treat most problems, if you are willing to make small compromises in dose homogeneity.

Suppose, in order to improve homogeneity and remain within critical constraints, you desire, say, a 52° wedge or a 21° wedge? The following method may be used to approximate any combination which will simulate any wedge angle up to the maximum wedge angle available (usually 60°).[11]

In most cases, when two fields from the same treatment unit have the same size and have the same wedge factor, then the wedge angles are equal. Another way of saying this is that a given wedge angle corresponds to a unique wedge factor. If there were a 52° wedge for a given treatment unit, it would have a characteristic wedge factor. Wedge factors can be found roughly by interpolating among known wedge factors for the existing wedges for that machine. (You should do this graphically, and not with straight linear interpolation, since the wedge factor is not a linearly changing function of wedge angle.)

Suppose you wish to use a combination of a wedge and an open field to simulate a wedged field with a lesser wedge angle. To achieve this simulation you would use the equation:

$$WT_1 \cdot w_1 + WT_2 \cdot w_2 = WT_3 \cdot w_3$$

where WT_1 and W_1 are the weight and wedge factor for the existing wedge respectively, the subscript 2 refers to the open field, and the subscript 3 refers to the desired simulated wedged field. Obviously, $W_2 = 1.0$, since the wedge factor for an open field is always 1.0.

A second equation is $WT_1 + WT_2 = WT_3$, since we are using the sums of fields 1 and 2 to simulate field 3. Thus we could rewrite the above equation:

$$WT_1 \cdot w_1 + (WT_3 - WT_1) = WT_3 \cdot w_3$$

from which we solve for WT_1:

$$WT_1 (w_1 - 1) + WT_3 = WT_3 \cdot w_3$$
$$WT_1 (w_1 - 1) = WT_3 (w_3 - 1)$$

$$WT_1 = WT_3 \left(\frac{w_3 - 1}{w_1 - 1} \right)$$

where $WT_2 = WT_3 - WT_1$, and WT_3 is known.

Of course, a weighted isodose summation should be done with a computer, or otherwise you must check that the calculated weights actually produce an acceptable dose distribution.

Example 11.1:

Use an open field in combination with a 60° wedge (wedge factor 0.49) to simulate a 45° wedge (wedge factor 0.58), the resulting field having a weight of 1.0 (or 100).

$$WT_1 = WT_3 \left(\frac{w_3 - 1}{w_1 - 1} \right) = 1.0 \left(\frac{0.58 - 1}{0.49 - 1} \right) = \frac{0.42}{0.51} = 0.82 \ (or \ 82)$$
$$WT_2 = 1.0 - 0.82 = 0.18 \ (or \ 18)$$

Thus the 60° wedge would be used 82% of the time, and an open field the other 18% of the time. This was done with Clinac-4 fields, and the comparison is shown in Figure 11.22.

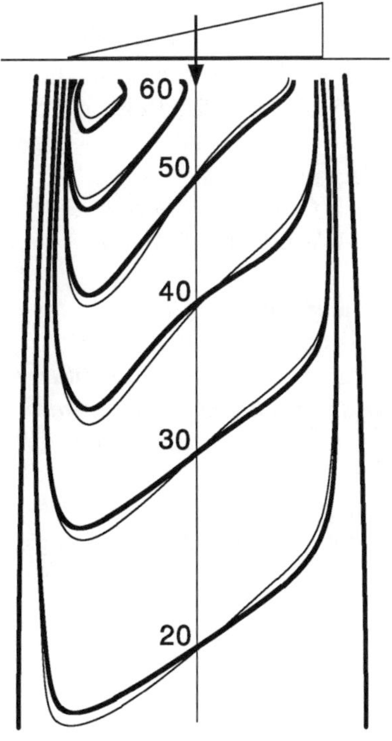

Figure 11.22. Solid lines represent isodose lines for a 6 x 8 cm field with a 45° wedge, Clinac-4. Dashed lines are computer generated isodose lines for an open 6 x 8 cm field with weight 18 combined with a 6 x 8 cm 60° wedge field with weight 82.

Example 11.2:

Use a 45° wedge and an open field to simulate a 22° wedged field having a weight of 0.5 (or 50). The wedge factor for a 22° wedged field for this treatment unit is 0.89, and for a 45° wedge, the wedge factor is 0.58.

$$WT_1 = WT_3 \left(\frac{w_3 - 1}{w_1 - 1}\right) = 0.5\left(\frac{0.89 - 1}{0.58 - 1}\right) = 0.5(0.26) = 0.13(or\ 13)$$
$$WT_2 = WT_3 - WT_1 = 0.5 - 0.13 = 0.37\ (or\ 37)$$

The weight for the 45° wedged field will be 13, and for the open field the weight will be 37.

References

1. Cohen, M., Burns, J.E., & Sears, R. "Physical Aspects Of Cobalt 60 Teletherapy Using Wedge Filters," *Acta Radiol* 53:401, 1960.
2. Tranter, F.W. "Design of Wedge Filters for Use with 4 MeV Linear Accelerator," *Br J Radiol* 30:329, 1957.
3. Van de Geijn, J. "A Simple Wedge Filter Technqiue for Cobalt 60 Teletherapy," *Br J Radiol* 35:710, 1962.
4. Aron, B.S. & Scapicchio, M. "Design of Universal Wedge Filter System for a Cobalt 60 Unit," *Am J Roent* 96:70, 1966.
5. Cohen, M. "Physical Aspects of Roentgen Therapy Using Wedge Filters," *Acta Radiol* 52:65 and 158, 1959; and 53:153, 1960.
6. Sonntag, A., Jordanow, D. & Bunde, E. "Wedge Filters in Cobalt 60 Teletherapy," *Electromedica* 3:65, 1968.
7. Van Rosenbeck, E., & Grimm, J. "Wedge Filters Their Construction Use with a 22 MeV Betatron," *American Journal of Roentgenology* 85:926, 1961.
8. Johns, H.E. & Cunningham, J.R. *The Physics of Radiology*, 4th Edition, Charles C. Thomas, 1985, pp. 396-397.
9. *Determination of Absorbed Dose ina Patient Irradiated by Beams of X or Gamma Rays in Radiotherapy Procedures*, Report 24, International Commission on Radiation Units, Washington, D.C., 1976, pp. 12-14.
10. Aron and Scapicchoi, pp. 12-14.
11. Zwicker, R.D., Shahabi, S., Wu, A., & Sternick, E.S. "Effective Wedge Angles for 6 - MV Wedges," *Med Phys* 12(3), 1985, pp. 347-349.

Irregularly Shaped Fields

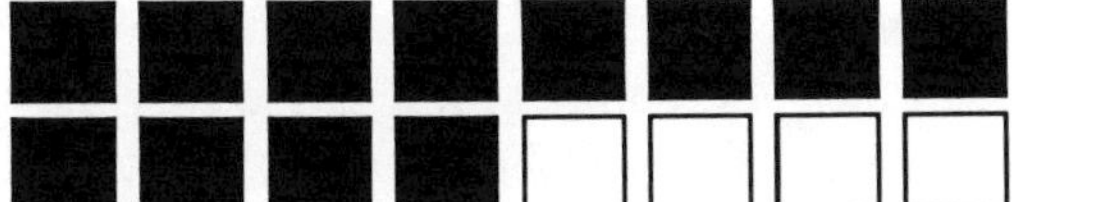

12

A. Shadow Tray
B. Field Shaping Blocks
C. The Effect of Blocking on Dosimetry Calculations
D. Estimating Dose in Shielded Areas (Block Shadows)
E. Treatment Duration with Shadow Tray

Not all tumor volumes are rectangular.

Nearly all therapy unit collimators, however, provide only square or rectangular fields. Older treatment units provided circular fields, and a few manufacturers have made collimators with small tungsten "fingers" which block the field and make its shape irregular. These have proven cumbersome, inadequate, heavy, and expensive. There is an easier way of creating irregularly shaped fields.

A.
Shadow Tray

Most treatment units can now accept a **shadow tray** or a blocking tray, a flat support made of acrylic, polycarbonate, or wire mesh which slides into a slot that positions the tray in the beam perpendicular to the central ray. This slotted support for the shadow tray may be permanently mounted on the collimator or it may be removable.

The presence of the shadow tray in the path of the beam may have an effect on the dose rate or monitor factor, since it removes some of the radiation by absorption and scatter, especially if the tray is made of plastic. Wire mesh may have some effect, but in most cases it is too small to take into account. You should verify this yourself and not assume it.

The **tray factor** is the radiation received at a normal treatment distance with the tray in place, divided by the radiation received under identical conditions, but without the tray in place (open field). The tray factor depends on many variables; the nature of the radiation, the thickness and composition of the tray, the field size, the source to tray distance, and the tray to patient distance. For a given treatment unit, the nature of the radiation and the source to tray distance are normally fixed, but the other factors are variable. The nature and composition of the tray may, as stated earlier, be either wire mesh, acrylic (Perspex, Plexiglas, Lucite), polycarbonate (Lexan), or it may be a combination of acrylic and leaded glass that will reduce skin dose. Each of these trays will have a different tray factor, which itself varies somewhat with field size and the position of the tray. A single tray factor with field size and position is averaged, and a single tray factor is usually used for a given tray. However, this is not good practice, since the tray factor varies by approximately $\pm 2\%$ with field size.

B.
Field Shaping Blocks

The shadow tray is designed to enable you to create shadows where the radiation is blocked out. This is done by placing absorbing blocks in the radiation field. These blocks may be of lead, tungsten, or a high density, low melting alloy[1] (e.g. Lipowitz's metal, Rose's metal).* The blocks may be part of a permanent inventory of standard sizes and shapes, or they may be custom made for an individual patient. The low melting point alloys are particularly suited to this, but custom blocks may be made with lead or lead shot with somewhat greater difficulty.

How thick should the blocks be? That is, what fraction of the radiation should be allowed to reach the patient? This is partly a matter of individual choice, and it is partly determined by how much room is available between the shadow tray and the bottom of the collimator. Normally the transmission factor is between 2% and 5%.

If the blocks are part of a permanent inventory, another problem arises. The blocks will probably have straight sides, whereas the rays of a radiation beam diverge.

In order to achieve a uniformly diminished beam in the shadow region, the blocks have to have sloping sides[2] (see Figure 12.2). The degree of slope depends on the displacement of the block from the central ray. The direction of slope depends on which side of the field is to receive the block. Thus an inventory of permanent blocks with different sloping sides is not practical.

---

* Lipowitz's metal, frequently referred to by one of its trade names, Cerrobend, is a low-melting point alloy composed of lead (26.7%), bismuth (50%), tin (13.3%), and cadmium (10%). The melting point is 70°C, well below the melting point of the individual components. Rose's metal is composed of lead, bismuth, and tin.

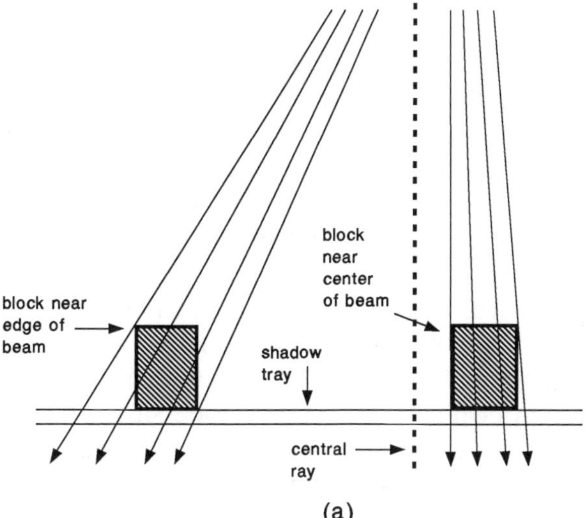

Figure 12.1. Straight sided blocks.

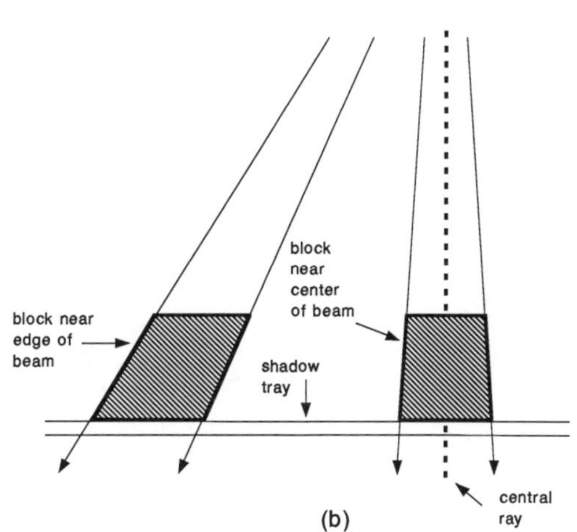

Figure 12.2. Diverging blocks.

The usual approach to getting around this impracticality follows.

(1) The patient is radiographed in what is to be the treatment position. The distance from the radiographic x-ray target to the skin is the same as the SSD to be used in treatment, and the central ray is anatomically the same in both cases. The radiographic field need not be limited to the therapy field. The source to film distance is carefully recorded.

(2) The therapist sketches on the radiograph the shadow pattern desired using visible anatomy and not the size of the area as a guide, since the images are magnified on the radiograph.

(3) The film is now positioned under a hot wire device, as pictured in Figure 12.3.[3,4] The distance from the pivot point of

the hot wire to the film must be the same as the target-film distance, and the suspension point must be vertically above the central ray mark on the film. A block of styrofoam plastic is positioned above the film so that its lower edge is the same distance from the hot wire pivot as the distance from the therapy source to the shadow tray.

(4) The lower end of the hot wire normally terminates in a stylus-like device which is slowly traced along the block-markings on the film. Fast motion will distort the wire. The wire cuts through the styrofoam in a pattern similar to the diverging rays which will bound the block in the treatment room. The cut-out section of styrofoam will thus have the degree and amount of slope required of the blocks in the treatment field and will be of the proper size to cast the correct shadow on the patient.

(5) The styrofoam block, minus the cutout section, is placed on a flat surface. The voids are filled to the proper thickness with an alloy with a low melting point such as Lipowitz's metal or Roses' metal. This material in molten form will not burn or melt the styrofoam.

Figure 12.3.
(a) Simulator room.
(b) Mold room.
(c) Treatment room.

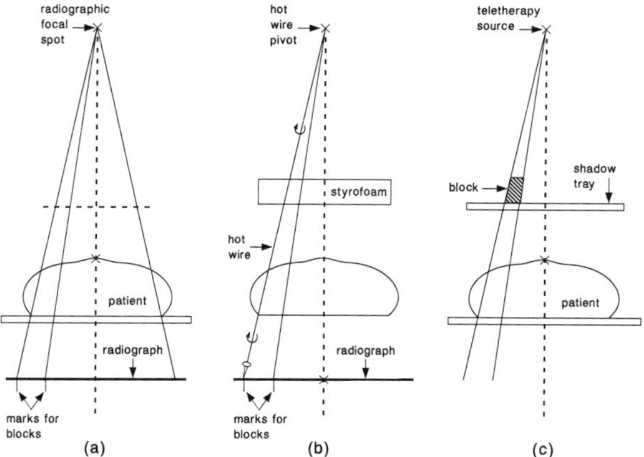

When the metal has cooled and solidified, the blocks are removed from the styrofoam ready for use. A radiographic check is normally performed to ensure the absence of any air cavity before the blocks are used for treatment. When the patient has completed his or her treatment, the blocks are melted down for reuse.

C.
The Effect of Blocking on Dosimetry Calculations

Since the blocks prevent a portion of the primary radiation from reaching the patient, the amount of scattered radiation reaching any specific point in the tissue is also reduced. Since scattered radiation is responsible for a significant fraction of the dose to all points, blocking has a profound effect on dosimetry calculations.

There is currently no exact way of taking the reduction of scattering into account.

Computer techniques using some form of the algorithmic such as **Clarkson method** give perhaps the best approximation.[5,6,7] The Clarkson method is certainly not suited to hand calculations; while it is relatively simple, it involves many steps and is extremely time consuming.

Many computer programs based on the Clarkson method utilize quantities called scatter-air ratios (SAR). Suppose you have a complete table of tissue air ratios (TAR) for circular fields. The table would consist of columns of TAR's, each column corresponding to a certain field radius and the number in the column being TAR's for that field size at various depths. A column for a zero radius field would be included. If you now subtract the TAR for the zero radius field at each depth from each of the TAR's for other field radii, you would have a new table whose values represent that portion of each TAR which was due to scatter, since the difference between two TAR's at the same depth is a difference due to scattered radiation.

We call this new table a table of scatter air ratios. Each value is calculated as follows:

$$SAR_x = TAR_x - TAR_o$$

where x is the radius of a circular field. We might similarly generate a table of scatter-maximum ratios (SMR) from a table of TMR's, but its generation would be complicated by the presence of ratios of the monitor factors.

Consider now the following "pie-slice":

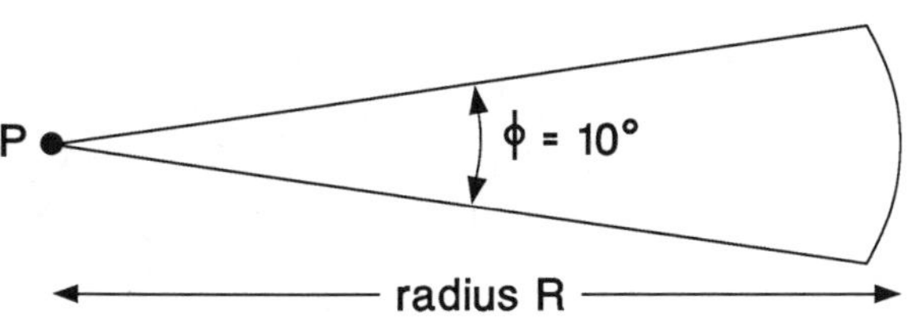

If we combine this with 35 similar slices, we would have a complete circle of radius R, with the point P at its center. (Each pie slice describes an angle of 10°, and there are 360° in a circle). If the circle thus formed represents a circular radiation field at some depth in tissue, then the point P will receive 1/36 as much scattered radiation from each 10° pie slice as it would receive from the entire circular field.

Now consider the following rectangular field with four blocks as in Figure 12.5:

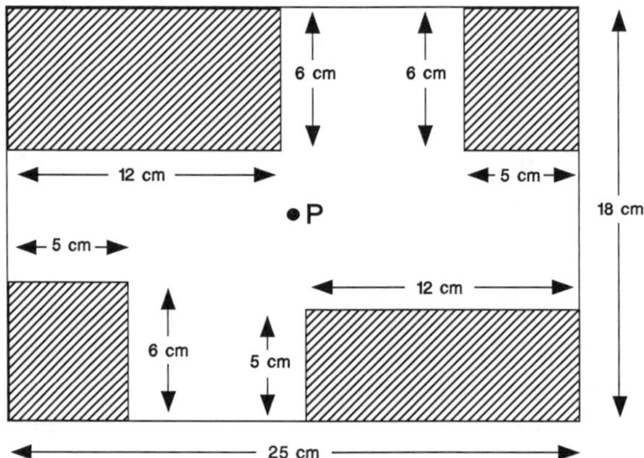

What is the depth dose fraction, TMR, or TAR at some depth (say 10 cm) below point P in this field? The following technique gives us an answer to this question for any depth below any point in the field.

We first draw in radials at 10° intervals from the point P to the edge of the field (or the edge of a block) as it is demonstrated in Figure 12.6.

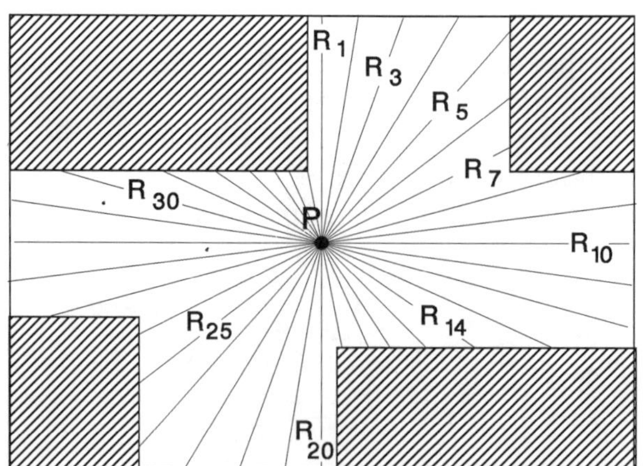

Each of these radials can be thought of as the centerline of a "pie slice." Below is a representation of the radial marked R_4 as shown in Figure 12.7, removed and enlarged from Figure 12.6:

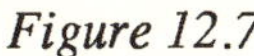

Figure 12.7

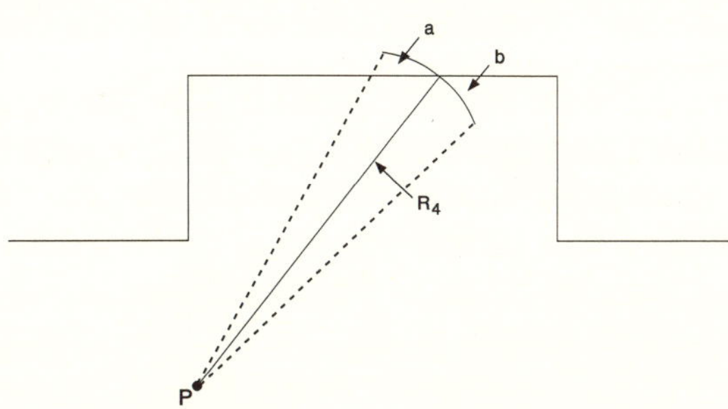

The small areas marked a and b are approximately the same size and roughly equidistant from point P, so the actual scatter from area b which is not included in the pie slice is closely compensated for by scatter from area a, if it were in the field.

In Figure 12.8, if we consider the entire blocked field to be composed of such pie slices, we would see it as a computer sees it when it uses the Clarkson technique.

Figure 12.8. Illustration of the Clarkson technique.

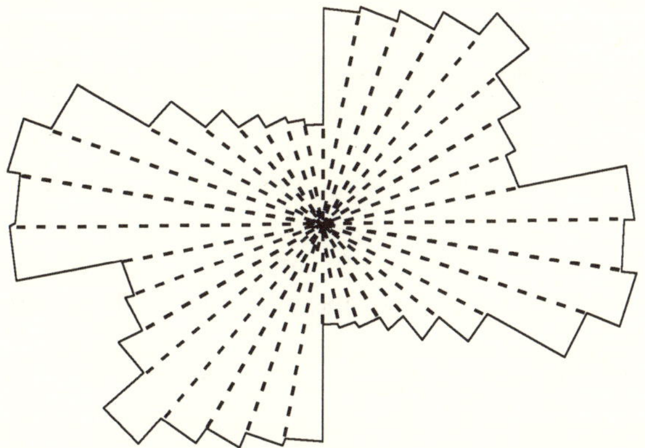

If we look up the SAR for any single radial for a circular field of that radius and divide by 36, we would have the scatter contribution to the TAR at that point due to the single pie slice corresponding to that radial. If we sum this contribution for all radials and add in the primary contribution, we will have the TAR at point P. From this, we can calculate the TMR, TPR, or ddf if we know the geometry involved.

Using a computer you could do this calculation at several hundred points within the field in minutes. To do so by hand would take a considerable length of time.

For the field pictured in Figure 12.5, assuming we are using a cobalt-60 unit, the depth dose fraction at 10 cm depth is found by the Clarkson method to be 0.608. Looking at the 80 cm depth dose tables, you see that this corresponds to an equivalent square of 14.94 cm. There are several "quick and dirty" methods of approximating equivalent squares for irregular fields:

(a) You can ignore the presence of the blocks. Obviously, this is an error and the greater the shadow area, the greater the error. In our example, this gives an equivalent square of 2 (18 x 25) / (18 + 25) = 20.93 cm, with a ddf of 0.636, a 4.6% error.

(b) You can lump all unblocked areas together as a square and assume the equivalent square side to be the square root of this area. This ignores elongations. The greater the elongation, the greater the error. In our example, the unblocked area is the square root of 258 cm^2, so the equivalent square by this method is the square root of 258 cm^2 = 16.06 cm. The corresponding ddf is 0.616, a 1.3% error.

(c) You can find the equivalent square of a rectangle whose sides are the length and average width of the largest single uninterrupted run. In our example, this would be 25 cm and about 7.5 cm, for an equivalent square of 11.54 cm, corresponding to a depth dose fraction of 0.585 (3.8%). This method ignores the scatter contribution of a significant portion of the unblocked area, yet it was recommended in the early days of dosimetry for Hodgkin's disease.

(d) You can use the unblocked field in calculations. Since our formula for equivalent square of a rectangular square field is 4 times area divided by perimeter (i.e., 2ab / (a + b) = 4ab / 2 (a + b), why not use area of unblocked field divided by perimeter of blocked field, and multiply by 4? In our example, this gives:

$$4 \ (258 \ cm^2 \ / \ 86 \ cm) = 12 \ cm$$

corresponding to a ddf of 0.593, a 2.5% error.

(e) You can approximate a rectangle having the same area as the unblocked portion of the field while essentially retaining the elongation. This is done as follows:

(1) Find the total shadow area (in this example, 180 cm^2).

(2) Divide this area by the length of that dimension of the field least affected by the blocking (in this case, 25 cm).

(3) Subtract this from the other dimension of the field (the dimension most affected), in this case 18 cm. 18 cm - 7.2 cm = 10.8 cm.

(4) Consider the equivalent square of the rectangle 10.8 x 25 cm which, in this case would be 15.08 cm, corresponding

to a ddf of 0.608, the same ddf found using the Clarkson method, i.e., a negligible error. Figure 12.9 will help you visualize this method.

Figure 12.9

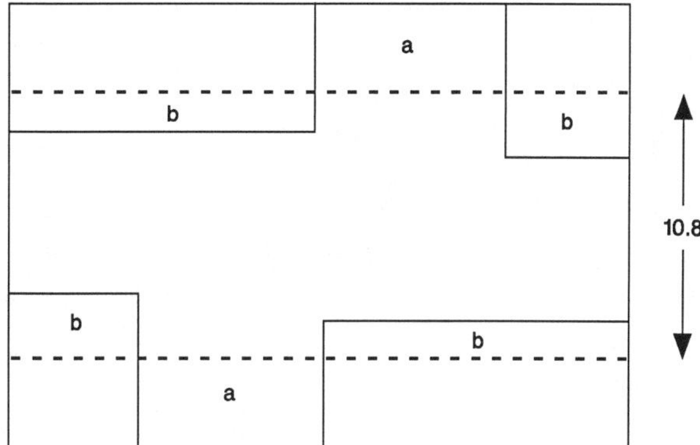

The areas marked (a) are in the field, but considered not to be in the equivalent rectangle; the areas marked (b) are not in the field, but are considered to be in the equivalent rectangle. The method assumes the total of (a) to be equal to the total of (b).

All of the above methods only give an estimate of an equivalent square. You must then use this information in some way to obtain a ddf or TMR. But where is this ddf or TMR most valid? Not necessarily in the center of the field, since in some cases, this point may lie in the shadow of a block. TMR or ddf is most valid in the centroid of the unblocked field, which is the approximate center of scatter of the remaining portion of the field, shifted by the presence of shadows. While the centroid can be found exactly using mathematical techniques, it would be foolish to apply them, since all of the above dimensions are approximations.

To estimate dose on rays other than the centroid, only the Clarkson method will give satisfactory answers.

D.
Estimating Dose in Shielded Areas (Block Shadows)

The Clarkson technique works outside the field as well as inside. Figure 12.10 shows point P lying outside the field. The same technique works for a point in the shadow of a block.

For the single pie slice shown in Figure 12.10, the scattered radiation at point P will be 1/36 of the scatter from a circular field of radius R_2, minus 1/36 of the scatter from a circular field of radius R_1, the segment in shadow. Performing similar

Figure 12.10

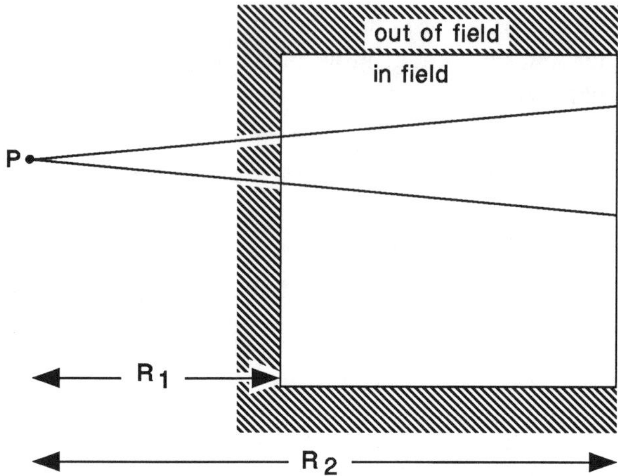

calculations for the other pie slices and adding in the primary radiation gives the TAR at point P. The primary contribution depends on the transmission through the collimator or on the block. A typical transmission is about 0.03.

As in the case of points within the field, the Clarkson technique proves too time consuming for hand calculation; a faster method is needed.

Simply saying that the dose in the shadow is equal to the radiation transmitted through the collimator or block is definitely wrong. Most of the dose here is due to scatter from the unblocked points of the field, and if the block is small this contribution is considerable.

For example, consider the dose 10 cm below point Q in Figure 12.5. The percentage of primary radiation penetrating to depth of 10 cm for a cobalt-60 beam at 80 cm SSD is 42.7%. (See Johns and Cunningham, p. 744, Table B-2, 0 x 0 cm field size).[8] If the block transmits 3% of the primary radiation, then the primary contribution to a ddf at this point is 0.03 x .427 = 0.013, or only 1.3% of the maximum dose along the central ray (D_{max}).

A Clarkson calculation for this point indicates that the contribution to the ddf due to scatter is 0.061, so the total ddf is 0.074, or 7.4% of the D_{max}, most of which is due to scatter.

Now let's try an approximation. First you must find the ddf without the presence of the blocks. We will use method (e) to find the equivalent square to be 17.28 cm with a corresponding ddf of 0.619. This would be the ddf at the centroid of the field; we will compensate for the fact that point Q is near the edge of the field after we assume the block is in place.

From this 0.619 value, we remove the ddf for a field whose size and position is that of our block, 6 x 12 cm, with an equivalent square of 8.0 cm, and a corresponding ddf of 0.552. This removes the primary radiation and that portion of the scatter in the blocked region.

Removing the ddf, we obtain a value of 0.067, for the scattered portion of ddf, compared to 0.061 from the Clarkson calculation. This estimate is a little high because the 0.619 is the ddf at the centroid of the unblocked field, whereas point Q is toward the edge. This error in a shielded area is not serious. To summarize:

(1) Using approximation method (e), find the equivalent square of the unblocked field, without considering the block whose shadow contains the point in question. From this, obtain the ddf at the depth of interest.

(2) Find the ddf at this depth for a field size equal to the block shadow. Subtract this from the ddf of step (1).

(3) If the block is near the centroid, make no correction. If it is near the edge of the field, multiply the result by 0.9 to reduce error.

(4) Add to this last step the primary radiation contribution, which is the product of the block transmission factor times the ddf for a very small field, nearly at the depth of interest.

E.
Treatment Duration with Shadow Tray

Our general formula for calculating treatment duration now looks like one of the following:

(1)   For SSD planning:

$$T = \frac{D_{pc} \cdot weight}{I_p \cdot w \cdot CAL \cdot N_c \cdot K_s}$$

(2)   For SAD planning:

$$T = \frac{D_{pc} \cdot weight}{I_p \cdot w \cdot TMR \cdot CAL \cdot N_c \cdot K_s}$$

where D_{pc} is prescription dose per cycle time; I_p is the isodose line chosen for prescription dose (or ddf, in the case of simple dosimetry); w is the wedge factor, where pertinent; N_c is the number of times this field is applied per cycle; K_s is the shadow tray factor (transmitted fraction); and CAL is a measure of output in a maxiphantom. If the tabulated output is measured in a

miniphantom, modify the expressions as follows:
(1) for SAD planning, replace TMR by TAR;
(2) for SSD planning, multiply CAL by PSF or BF. If the tabulated output is in terms of exposure, it must also by multipled by the f-factor. For each of the variables which depend on field size, you must decide what field size to use when looking them up:
(a) For the variable which depends on depth (DDF, I_p, TMR, TAR, or TPR) and if used, for the scatter factor (PSF or BF), you should use the effective field size as calculated in this chapter, i.e., the equivalent square of the unblocked portion of the blocked field.
(b) For the output (CAL), you should use the equivalent square of the collimator setting, i.e. the size you would get before blocks are added. This is only an approximation for the cases where output is measured in a maxipahntom; it should be corrected by multiplying CAL by the ratio of PSF for the two field sizes. The correction is close to one for high energies, and the usual practice is to ignore it. For cobalt-60 energies and lower, the output is usually measured in a miniphantom.

References

1. Powers, W.E., Kinzie, J.J., Demidecki, A.J., Bradfield, J.S., & Feldman, A. "A New System of Field Shaping for External-Beam Radiation Therapy," *Radiology* 108:407, 1973.
2. Kuisk, H. "New Method to Facilitate Radiotherapy Planning and Treatment, Including a Method for Fast Production of Solid Lead Blocks with Diverging Walls for Cobalt 60 Beam," *Am J Roentgenol* 117:161, 1973.
3. Edland, R.W. & Hansen, H. "Irregular Field-Shaping for Cobalt 60 Teletherapy," *Radiology* 92:1567, 1969.
4. Jones, D. "A Method for the Accurate Manufacture of Lead Shields," *Br J Radiol* 44:398, 1971.
5. Clarkson, J. "A Note on Depth Doses in Fields of Irregular Shape," *Br J Radiol*, 14:265, 1941.
6. Johns, H.E. & Cunningham, J.R. *The Physics of Radiology*, 4th Edition, Charles C. Thomas, 1983, pp. 344-346, 374-376.
7. Cunningham, J.R. "Scatter-Air Ratios," *Phys Med Biol* 17:42, 1972.
8. Johns & Cunningham, p. 744.

Arc Therapy

13

A. *Simulating the Lens Effect*
B. *Isodose Summation in Arc Therapy*
C. *The Effect of Blocking on Dosimetry Calculations*
D. *Calculation of Treatment Duration in Arc Therapy*
E. *Arc Therapy Planning Without a Computer*

You probably at one time or other in your childhood burned a dead leaf by concentrating the rays of the sun through a simple magnifying lens. You do this by holding the lens perpendicular to the sun's rays and moving it up and down until the bright spot is as small as possible on the leaf; only then will it begin to smoke. You may then have experimented on your own hand. When the bright spot was small, it smarted fiercely; but when you moved the lens closer so that the bright spot got larger, the spot was only slightly warm. What you were doing was gathering all the energy on the lens surface and applying it to a very small area, so that the energy per square centimeter increased greatly.[1]

Why isn't this same principle used in treating cancer patients with ionizing radiation? Unfortunately, the principle of light refraction by lenses does not apply to high energy radiation. We cannot bend x- and gamma rays with a lens.

A.
Simulating the Lens Effect

Figure 13.1 shows how to accomplish the same effect as a lens, not by bending the rays, but by changing the position of the source during treatment.

Concentrating radiation at a point can be done by using a number of fixed fields, or by using an infinite number of fields spaced an infinitesimal distance apart, rotating the source smoothly and continuously around the isocenter while delivering radiation. This is called arc therapy.

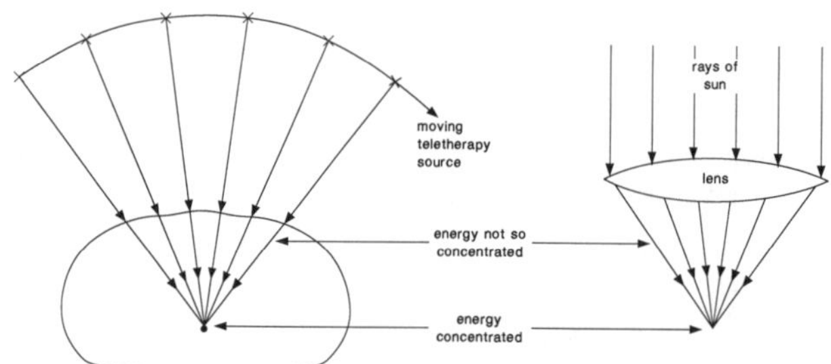

*Figure 13.1.
Similarity between
arc therapy and
lens function.*

Since the field is always directed at the isocenter, but passes only briefly through surface tissues, the dose to the isocenter is maximized. The isocenter corresponds loosely to the focal point of a lens, while the tissues close to the surface correspond to your hand held close to the lens, where the rays are not concentrated.

The arc of the source during treatment may measure anywhere from 50° to 60° to a complete 360° rotation. The greater the arc, the less the actual dose to subcutaneous tissues.   On the other hand, with a greater arc, a greater amount of tissue receives some dose. Arc therapy is limited by the high integral dose associated with it.

B.
Isodose Summation in Arc Therapy

Isodose distributions for arc therapy techniques could be obtained by either measurement or calculation. In-phantom measurements were performed using many small ion chambers.[2,3] Calculations of arc distributions are based on the superposition of many single beam isodose distributions.

Obviously, it would take infinite time to sum the isodose lines from an infinite number of fields. Fortunately, a very good approximation is obtained by summing the contributions of a large number of closely spaced fields, for example, 10° apart. The closer the spacing, the better the approximation.

To do this for even a half circle arc (180°) would require the summing of 18 isodose maps. You should do this by hand at least once so that you understand the complexity of the process. The complexity is one reason why the use of arc therapy is not more widespread. In precomputer days, not so very long ago, people realized that arc therapy offered great advantages, but they could never be very sure of the resulting dose distribution. The advent of fast computers should have caused a great interest in the technique, but therapists had grown accustomed to using 3 and 4 field techniques for certain treatments, and often simply didn't consider arc therapy in cases where it might have been the optimum treatment method.

The isodose patterns in Figure 13.2 were computer generated. Notice in Figure 13.2 that the isodose curves are not circular, but slightly elliptical. Furthermore, the major axis of the isodose ellipses are perpendicular to the major axis (longest dimension) of the ellipse of the body. This orientation is a natural consequence of the fact that the radiation can more easily penetrate the thinner portion of the body (the minor axis) and thus the high dose region extends closer to the surface along this axis.

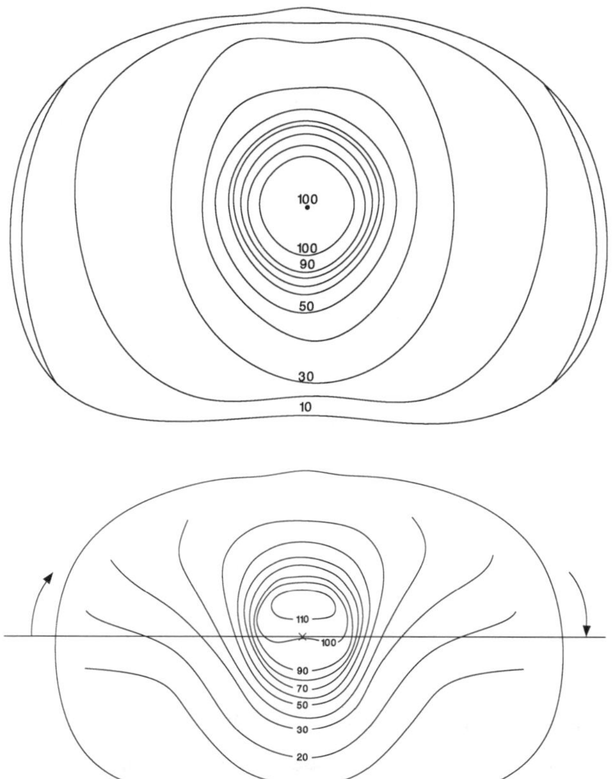

Figure 13.2. 360° rotational therapy using a 7 x 9 cm field on a 4 MV linear accelerator.

Figure 13.3. 180° rotational therapy using a 7 x 9 cm field on a 4 MV linear accelerator.

Figure 13.3 demonstrates the isodose distribution resulting from semicircular arc. The highest dose region is shifted anteriorly, so that some past pointing is required. This is true of all partial arcs.

Observe also that the entire summation is normalized at the isocenter, i.e., the value of the isodose line passing through isocenter has the value 100 or 1.0. In the past, when using more than one beam, the isodose value at isocenter has been the total weight of all beams used. If we considered an arc to have an infinite number of beams, the value at isocenter would be infinite.

Instead we normalize as if only one beam is in use. This will be true in calculating treatment duration as well.

In the case of the 120° arc (Fig. 13.4), hot spots tend to be located above the axis. Both here and in the last summation, values in excess of 100 are located in the hot spot. The subcutaneous dose increases as the arc becomes smaller.

Figure 13.4. 120° rotational therapy using a 7 x 9 cm field on a 4 MV linear accelerator.

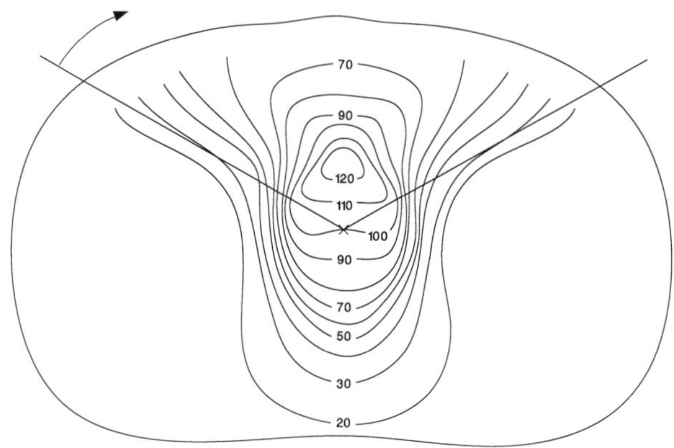

Figure 13.5. Anterior-posterior opposed pair of 120° arcs on a 4 MV linear accelerator, 7 x 9 cm field.

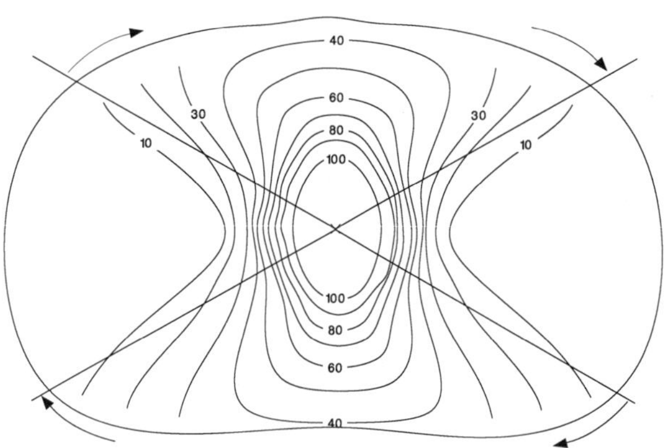

With two separate opposing arcs (Fig. 13.5), similar to opposing beams, we eliminate the necessity of past pointing, and also gain the advantage of passing the beam through only the relatively thin portions of the patient; however, the tendency toward elliptical isodose curves is increased.

Treatment using two separate arcs may sometimes be accomplished with a technique called skip scanning. Some treatment units may be programmed to turn the beam off and on in specific portions of a continuous arc. More often, however, this capability does not exist, and the two arcs must be separately planned and executed. The dose summation is accomplished the same in either case, the advantage of skip scanning being a reduction of time in the treatment room.

Double or multiple arc techniques are also employed to avoid overdosing critical structures such as the spinal cord, rectum, etc. Figure 13.6 shows a typical summation of a two arc technique used in treatment of the prostate.

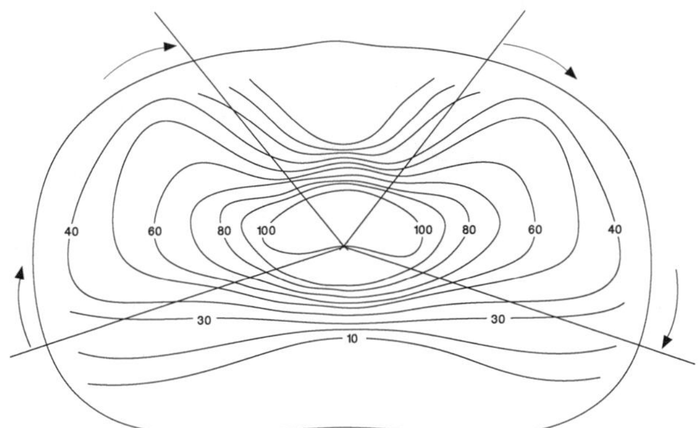

Figure 13.6. Two 70° lateral arcs on a 4 MV linear accelerator, 7 x 9 cm field.

C.

The Effect of Blocking on Dosimetry Calculations

We may use the same equation that we developed for a single SAD beam:

$$T = \frac{D_{pc} \cdot weight}{TMR \cdot w \cdot CAL \cdot I_p \cdot N_c \cdot K_s}$$

which simplifies in most cases to:

$$T = \frac{D_p}{TMR \cdot CAL \cdot I_p}$$

since for arc therapy the cycle time is normally one day, there is no wedge, and there is no shadow tray.

The TMR (or TAR) in the above equation is a single value corresponding to the average skin to isocenter distance, averaged over an arc whose characteristics will be discussed in the section on hand calculation. If a computer has done the isodose summation, it will provide you with this average skin to isocenter distance, or with appropriate TMR or TAR.

In addition to treatment duration, the treatment station technologist will require different set-up instructions from those for single fields, since the field is continuously in motion on the skin during treatment. Instructions for locating the isocenter, value of the start angle, value of the stop angle, and rate of rotation should be part of the dosimetry workup.

Rate of rotation may be specified as (1) degrees per minute in the case of constant output devices such as cobalt-60 units (i.e., when treatment duration is specified as a time rather than an integrated monitor setting), or as (2) a number of monitor units per degree. For example, in the case of cobalt-60 units:

$$degrees/minute = \frac{total\ arc}{treatment\ time}$$

or in the case of linear accelerators:

$$\mu/degree = \frac{(treatment\ duration\ in\ \mu)}{total\ arc}$$

D.
Calculation of Treatment Duration in Arc Therapy

No isodose summation is used in arc therapy done without a computer. While isodose summation by hand is possible, it is not usually practical because of the time involved. However, dose values to individual critical points can be readily found and the dose to the isocenter must be found in order to calculate treatment duration.

To obtain dose values, the first step is to lay out a polar coordinate system on the patient contour, with origin at the isocentric axis (Figure 13.7).

Figure 13.7. Polar representation of the patient contour, arc angle of 15°.

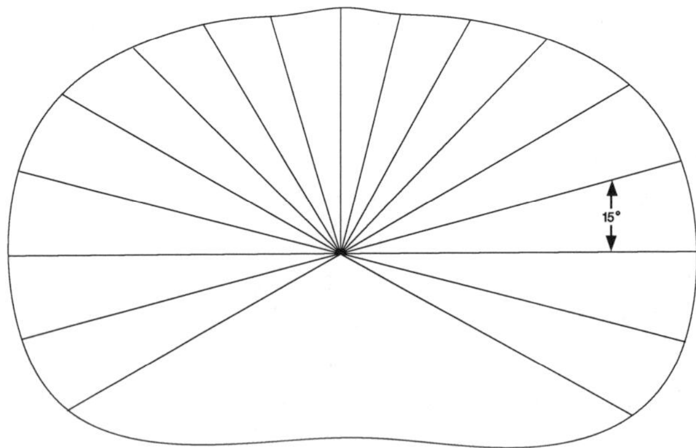

Radials are drawn from the axis to the skin at regular intervals. The angle between radials used is a matter of personal choice. Remember that the smaller the angle, the more radials, and the more accurate is the calculation. An angle separation of 15°, as shown in the figure, is usually sufficient.

These radials are laid out spanning the proposed arc, such as the 240° arc as in Figure 13.7. The length of each radial is measured. Now two approaches are possible. For each radial, you could obtain a TMR for that depth from a TMR table and then average the TMR's. Or you could average the lengths of the radials and look up a single TMR for that depth. TMR is used in the example, but you could use TAR or TPR, depending on the nature of the calibration (CAL).

The first calculation involves more work and theoretically is more accurate, but in practice no appreciable difference exists between the values obtained from the first and second methods.

Actually, you do not simply average the lengths of the radials. For greater accuracy, you must treat the outermost radials corresponding to the starting angle and stopping angle as half-weight radials. The reason for this is that the beam begins moving while its central ray is on this radial. As the unit rotates, only half the beam passes through this radial. The same is true at the last radial, where the beam stops with its central ray on the radial, with only half the field passing the radial. All other radials experience irradiation from the entire field. Since the penumbra approaches the radial from one side, the entire beam sweeps past the radial and then leaves it via its penumbra on the other side of the field.

In summary, you measure all radials, average the two end radials, and then add this average to the lengths of all other radials. You then divide this number by the total number of length you have added (which is one less than the number of radials you measured).

Whichever approach is used, the result is called an average TMR. We will write this as TMR_{ave} to denote this.

If you consider the dose to the isocenter to be the prescription dose, treatment duration is given by:

$$T = \frac{D_p}{TMR_{ave} \cdot CAL}$$

At this point, however, no reference is made to an actual target volume or to a dose at its boundary. The simplicity of the above equation is based on the fact that, by definition, the isodose value at the axis is 100% (or 1.0). The dose at the boundary of the desired target volume might be 85%, and there may be a partial volume where the dose is 115%, especially if we are dealing with a partial arc. This is why an isodose summation is highly desirable.

Short of a complete isodose summation, point by point calculation at critical points other than the isocenter can aid in decision making. A point calculation at one spot on the boundary of the target volume or a point within a critical structure will yield valuable information. A procedure for obtaining calculations at critical points appears below.

A properly sized single field isodose chart which has been normalized at the isocenter for SAD planning is needed. Also required is a TMR for each individual radial for the depth corresponding to the skin-isocenter distance for that radial.

Now you place the single field isodose map on the patient contour so that its central ray coincides with the first radial, and the normalization point (100%) is on the isocenter. You then read off the dose value at the point of interest. This may be zero if the beam does not pass through that point on a given radial. If the point lies within the beam, some visual interpolation between isodose lines is normally necessary, but this can be done quickly and with sufficient accuracy without resorting to a ruler and calculator. You now multiply the decimal value of the dose value you just obtained from your figure by the skin-isocenter TMR for that radial, and record the result.

This procedure is repeated for each of the radials. An average is taken of the adjusted TMR's. The isodose value at this point of interest is then the ratio of the result to the average TMR at the isocenter for a decimal value, multiplied by 100 for a percentage value.

This is a somewhat lengthy procedure. Once the contour has been marked off in radials and the individual TMR's obtained for each radial, you will spend at least 5 minutes per point. If a closely spaced grid of points is calculated in this manner, an isodose summation could be obtained. In essence, this is what the computer does.

References

1. Giancoli, D.C. *Physics Principles with Applications*, Prentice-Hall, 1980, Chapter 21.
2. Dahl, O. & Vikterlof, K.J. "Dose Distributions in Arc Therapy in the 200 to 250 KV Range," *Acta Radiol* [suppl.], Stockh 171, 1958.
3. Hultberg, S. et al. "Kilocurie Cobalt 60 Therapy at the Radiumhemmet," *Acta Radiol* [suppl.], Stockh 179, 1959.
4. Giancoli, D.C. *Physics Principles with Applications*, Prentice-Hall, 1980, Chapter 21.

Abutting Field Techniques

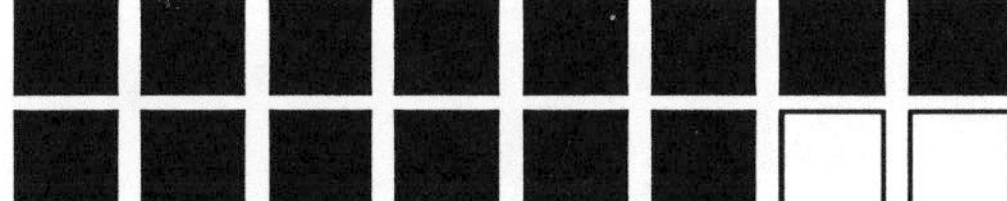

A. Divergence Overlap
B. Gapping Between Fields
C. Angling to Defeat Divergence
D. Opposing Pairs of Adjacent Fields
E. Frequent Errors with Adjacent Fields
F. Staggering the Gap (Moving Gap)

From time to time it is necessary to span the length of a target volume with more than one field.[1,2,3,4] There are many reasons for this, the most obvious of which is that the target volume is larger than the largest available field size.

Whatever the reason, unique problems arise when it becomes necessary to orient fields side by side.

A.
Divergence Overlap

Consider two fields aligned side by side with their central rays parallel (Figure 14.1).

If two field boundaries abut at the surface, they begin to overlap immediately below the surface, since each is diverging into the tissue treated by the other. This creates a normally unacceptable hot region between the fields.[5]

There are two basic approaches to this problem. One can either separate the fields slightly, leaving a gap between the boundaries, or one can angle the central rays away from each other so that the rays at the edges of the two fields are parallel and do not diverge into each other.[6] Both approaches are beset by their own peculiar disadvantages, as we shall see. Other techniques by which one can achieve dose uniformity across the junction is given elsewhere.[7-13]

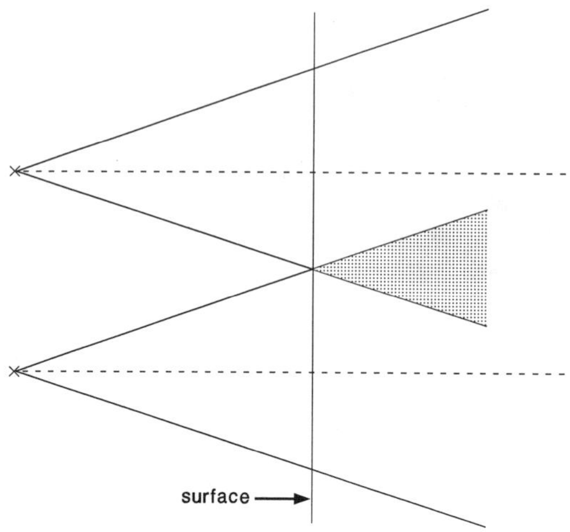

Figure 14.1. Geometric configuration of two adjacent beams abutting at the surface.

B.
Gapping Between Fields

Figures 14.2 through 14.5 illustrate the boundary region between two 20 x 20 cm Clinac-4 fields (80 cm SSD) with respectively a 0, 1, 2 and 3 cm gap.

One sees here that the hot spot does not disappear, but moves progressively deeper into the tissue, where the dose level eventually falls to below tissue tolerance. However, from the surface extending downward grows a "cold" region; i.e., a region of underdose which becomes more serious as the gap increases. Between the hot region and cold region is a region of relative homogeneity, where the target volume should be if this gapping technique is to be at all applicable. Actually, there is no region where the dose is perfectly homogeneous (no horizontal straight isodose line below the surface at any depth), because the isodose lines of the individual fields themselves are not flat.

Assuming that the gapping technique can be applied in a specific case (i.e., a cold spot can be tolerated above a certain depth, and a hot spot below), how great should the gaps between the fields be made?

Suppose we have a specification of a depth at which we require the closest approach to homogeneity. We also know the field sizes (widths A and B in the direction of adjacent alignment), and the SSD's (to keep the problem as general as possible, we allow different SSD's for the two fields, though in practice, they will normally be the same). Call the SSD's S_1 and S_2.

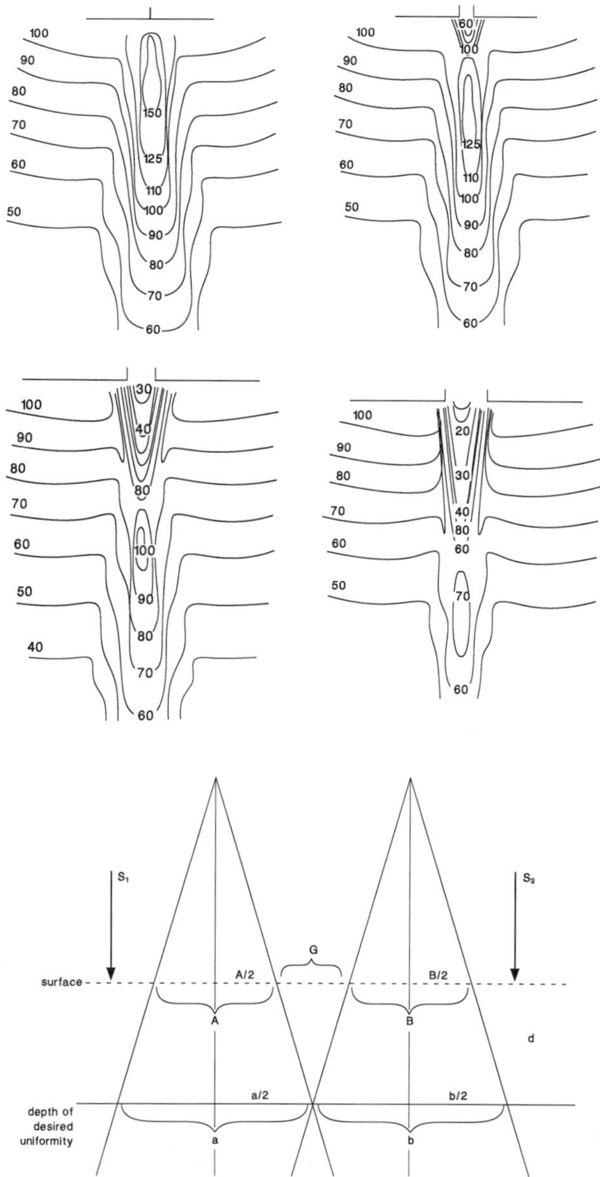

Figure 14.2. Dose distribution for two adjacent beams, 20 x 20 cm fields, 4 MV, Gap = 0 cm.

Figure 14.3. Dose distribution for two adjacent beams, 20 x 20 cm fields, 4 MV, Gap =1 cm.

Figure 14.4. Dose distribution for two adjacent beams, 20 x 20 cm fields, 4 MV, Gap = 2 cm.

Figure 14.5. Dose distribution for two adjacent beams, 20 x 20 cm fields, 4 MV, Gap =3 cm.

Figure 14.6. Two beams adjacent on the surface, separated by a distance G and matching at depth d.

We shall call the depth of desired homogeneity d, and assume that it will be the depth below the surface where the edges of the fields begin to overlap. We designate the gap between the field as G.

From the small rectangle formed between the two central rays and the surface and depth line, we see that the line A/2 + G + B/2 is the same length as the line a/2 + b/2. By equating the lengths, we obtain G:

$$G = \frac{a}{2} + \frac{b}{2} - \frac{A}{2} - \frac{B}{2} = \frac{1}{2}\left(a + b - A - B\right)$$

by property of similar triangles:

$$a = \left(\frac{S_1 + d}{S_1}\right) A \text{, and } b = \left(\frac{S_2 + d}{S_2}\right) B$$

By substituting a and b in the above expression for G we obtain:

$$G = \frac{1}{2}\left(\frac{S_1 + d}{S_1} A + \frac{S_2 + d}{S_1} B - A - B\right)$$

$$= \frac{A}{2}\left(\frac{S_1 + d}{S_1} - 1\right) + \frac{B}{2}\left(\frac{S_2 + d}{S_2} - 1\right)$$

$$= \frac{A}{2}\left(\frac{S_1 + d - S_1}{S_1}\right) + \frac{B}{2}\left(\frac{S_2 + d - S_2}{S_2}\right)$$

$$\textit{therefore, } G = \frac{d}{2}\left(\frac{A}{S_1} + \frac{B}{S_2}\right)$$

if both fields are at the same SSD ($S_1 = S_2 = S$), this simplifies to:

$$G = \frac{d}{2S}(A + B)$$

and in the special case where the fields sizes are equal ($A = B$) and have the same SSD ($S_1 = S_2 = S$):

$$G = \frac{Ad}{S}$$

With isocentric set-up, the form of equation is:

$$G = \frac{d}{2SAD}(A + B)$$

Example 14.1:

A field 20 cm wide with an SSD of 8 cm is to be aligned adjacent to a field 24 cm wide at 90 cm SSD. If maximum homogeneity is required at a depth of 8 cm, how much gap should be left between these fields at the surface?

$$G = \frac{Ad}{2S_1} + \frac{Bd}{2S_2} = \frac{20\ cm\ \times 8\ cm}{2 \times 80\ cm} + \frac{24\ cm\ \times 8\ cm}{2 \times 90\ cm} = \frac{160\ cm}{160} + \frac{192\ cm}{180} = 2.07\ cm$$

Example 14.2:

Repeat the above with both fields at 90 cm SSD.

$$G = \frac{d}{2S}(A + B) = \frac{8\ cm}{180}(24\ cm + 20\ cm) = 1.96\ cm$$

Example 14.3:

Repeat the above if both fields are 24 cm wide and both at 80 cm SSD.

$$G = \frac{Ad}{S} = 24 \cdot \left(\frac{8}{80}\right) = 2.4 \, cm$$

C.
Angling to Defeat Divergence

If the adjacent edges of the fields can be made parallel, the fields will neither diverge into each other or away from each other. Since the edge of the field angles away from the central ray, this can be accomplished by angling the central rays away from each other by an angle equal to the sum of the two field divergence angles (Figure 14.7); or stated another way, by angling each central ray away from the junction by the divergence angle of its respective fields.

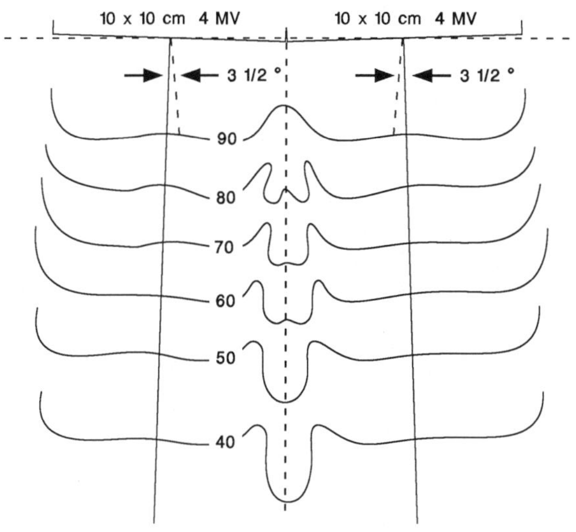

Figure 14.7. Abutting two fields by angling each central ray away from the junction.

The divergence angle of a field depends upon the field width and the SSD. A right triangle is formed by the central ray, edge of the field and half width of field at that SSD (Figure 14.8). The trigonometric function "tangent" of an angle is the ratio of the triangle leg opposite the angle in question divided by the leg adjacent to it, not the hypotenuse. In figure 14.8:

$$\tan \theta = \frac{A}{2SSD}$$

Figure 14.8

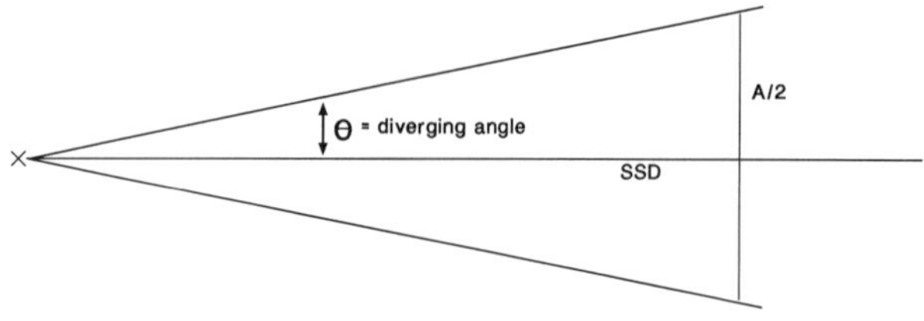

Thus we can say that θ is the angle whose tangent is A/(2 x SSD). Another way to write this is:

$$\theta = \tan^{-1} \frac{A}{2SSD}, \text{ or } \theta = Arctan \frac{A}{2SSD}$$

For calculating the angle θ you need either a calculator capable of calculating trigonometric functions, or a table of trigonometric functions. However, since you are likely to round off the angle to the nearest degree, the following table 14.1 will give the needed information.

Table 14.1: Diverging angle values for different SAD or SSD and various field sizes.

Div. Angle	SAD or SSD = 60	70	80
1°	3	3	3, 4
2°	4, 5	4, 5, 6	5, 6
3°	6, 7	7, 8	7, 8, 9
4°	8, 9	9, 10, 11	10, 11, 12
5°	10, 11	12, 13	13, 14, 15
6°	12, 13	14, 15	16, 17, 18
7°	14, 15	16, 17, 18	19, 20, 21
8°	16, 17	19, 20	22, 23
9°	18, 19, 20	21, 22, 23	24, 25, 26
10°	21, 22	24, 25	27, 28, 29
11°	23, 24	26, 27, 28	30, 31, 32
12°	25, 26	29, 30, 31	33, 34, 35
13°	27, 28	32, 33	36, 37, 38
14°	29, 30, 31	34, 35, 36	39, 40, 41
15°	32, 33	37, 38	42-44

90	100	110	120
3, 4	3-5	3-5	3-6
5-7	6-8	6-9	7-10
8-10	9-12	10-13	11-14
11-14	13-15	14-17	15-18
15-17	16-19	18-21	19-23
18-20	20-22	22-25	24-27
21-23	23-26	26-28	28-31
24-26	27-29	29-32	32-35
27-30	30-33	33-36	36-40
31-33	34-37	37-40	41-44
34-36	38-40	41-44	45-48
37-39	41-44	45-48	49-53
40-43	45-47	49-52	54-57
44-46	48-51	53-56	58-62
47-49	52-55	57-60	63-66

For example, if an 18 cm wide field at 80 cm is to be made adjacent to a 25 cm wide field at 100 cm (SSD or SAD), the 18 cm field is found under the 80 cm column in the 6° row; the 25 cm field is found under the 100 cm column in the 7° row; the central rays should be angled away from each other by 13°. It does not matter if they are angled 6° and 7° respectively, or if they are each angled 6.5° from the junction, or if one field is angled 13° and the other not at all.

A compound angle of more than 10° or 12° creates the problem of extra tissue irradiated at the outer boundaries of the fields. Also, such angling may be difficult or impossible in some cases with beam-stopper treatment units.

Another way to make the field edges parallel is to use a "half-beam block" which will block half of the field.

D.
Opposing Pairs of Adjacent Fields

The same schemes discussed for adjacent fields from one side can be used for opposing pairs, the major differences being in the case of gapped fields. Here, the "cold" spots of the junction from one side will overlap the "hot" spots from the opposite pair. These will not nearly compensate, but they will tend to broaden somewhat the region of approximate homogeneity.[14,15]

E.
Frequent Errors With Adjacent Fields

Aside from the error of omission of some compensating technique such as the two outlined above, there are some common errors which one should make a special effort to avoid.

One of these involves simulation of adjacent fields. Normal simulation cannot be trusted. This is because the target is moved with respect to the patient between views, changing the geometrical relationships. If a single radiograph is made, the individual fields will seem to overlap significantly on the radiograph, whereas the actual overlap in the patient may be slight or nonexistent.

What can be trusted is the relation of each fields' boundaries to the internal anatomy when the fields are viewed separately. This should be the criterion in judging the correctness of the set-up.

Another error involves a tendency on the part of treatment room technologists to direct a field perpendicularly to the surface. When different degrees of curvature are present on the surfaces to receive adjacent fields, this makes the angular relationship between the central rays of the two fields a matter of pot luck. If the surface is convex (like the exterior of a sphere), a serious hot spot will result; if the surface is concave (like the inner surface of a sphere), a cold spot may occur.

Once the first field is aligned to the patient, the second field must be aligned in accordance with the first field, not the patient. This is true whether you are using a gapping technique or an angling technique.

In most clinical set-ups, there is a vertabrae or other structure visible at the depth at which the matching takes place. Matching the fields at a structure is more reliable than skin gap techniques.

F.
Staggering the Gap (Moving Gap)

If you are using a gap technique, you have already decided to compromise to the extent of accepting hot or cold areas. These may be minimized over a period of several days by having the gap occur over a different skin area each fraction day for several days and then repeating the process clinically.[16]

As an example, suppose you have an area to be treated whose width at the surface is 36 cm. The depth and SSD are such that this can be done with two 17 cm fields separated by a gap of 2 cm. An alternative approach is to break the schedule up into (for example) three day cycles. On day one, fields A and B are respectively given widths of 15 and 19 cm with a 2 cm gap; on day two, 17 cm an 17 cm with a 2 cm gap; and on day three, 19 and 15 cm respectively, with a 2 cm gap; after which the cycle is repeated until the end of treatment.

The advantage of this is that the variation in dose between the homogeneous region and the hot or cold areas is now only 1/3 as great as it would be with a "stationary gap" routine. If the cycle chosen is four fractions rather than three, the variation would be approximately 1/4 as great, and so on. Observe, however, that the daily shift in the gap must be at least as great as the width of the gap itself. If the gap is to be 2 cm and a four day cycle is chosen, the variation in field sizes will have a range of at least 8 cm. This may not be feasible, since the probable reason for not using a single port to treat the problem was an inability to achieve a field size large enough. The required variation in field size to use the moving gap technique may also excess the field size limitations, if the cycle is too long.

The disadvantage of this method is the greatly increased complexity of the treatment schedule and set-up routine, with an accompanying increased chance for error.

References

1. Paterson, E. & Farr, R.F. "Cerebellar Medulloblastoma: Treatment by Irradiation of the Whole Central Nervous System," *Acta Radiological* 39:323-336, 1953.
2. Bloom, H.J.G., Wallace, E.N.K., Henk, J.M. "The Treatment and Prognosis of Medulloblastoma in Children," *Amer J of Roentgen* 105:43-62, 1969.
3. Bloom, H.J.G. "Concepts in the Natural History and Treatment of Medulloblastoma in Children: Increasing Survival Rates and Possible Risks with Current Radiotherapy Techniques," *CRC Critical Reviews in Radiological Sciences*, 2:89-143, 1971.
4. Jenkin, R.D.T. "Medulloblastoma in Childhood: Radiation Therapy," *Can Med Assoc J* 100:51-53, 1969.
5. Hopfan, S., Reid, A., Simpson, C., & Ager, P. "Clinical Complications Arising from Overlapping of Adjacent Radiation Fields: Physical and Technical Considerations," *Int J Radiation Oncology, Biol Phys* 2:801, 1977.
6. Bentel, G.C., Nelson, C.E., & Noell, K.T. *Treatment Planning & Dose Calculation in Radiation Oncology*, 3rd Edition, Pergamon Press, 1982, pp. 114-116.
7. Armstrong, D. & Tait, J. "The Matching of Adjacent Fields in Radiotherapy," *Radiology* 108:419-422, 1973.
8. Fraass, B.A., Tepper, J.E., Glatstein, E. & Van de Geijn, J. "Clinical Use of a Match-line Wedge for Adjacent Megavoltage Radiation Field Matching," *International Journal of Radiation Oncology, Biology, Physics* 9:209-216, 1983.
9. Wu, A., Sternick, E.S., Shahabi, S., Zwicker, R.D. "A Technique for Delivering Uniform Dose at the Junction of Two Spinal Fields," *British Journal of Radiology*, 59:929-930, 1986.
10. Doppke, K. "Treatment Strategies - Hodkin's Disease," in *Advances in Radiation Therapy Treatment Planning*. Wright, A.E. & Boyer, A.L., Eds. American Institute of Physics, New York, 1983, pp. 341-355.
11. Garavaglia, G. "Field Separation of Adjoining Therapy Fields," *Med Phys* 8:882, 1981.
12. Starchman, D.E., Leoffler, R.K., Sommer, R.D. "Achievement of Uniform Dose Without Overlap in Multi-Port Treatment Fields, Including Interport Shaped Blocks," *Radiology* 108:695 1973.
13. Griffin, T.W., Schumacher, D., Berry, H.C. "A Technique for Cranial-Spinal Irradiation," British Journal of Radiology 49:887-888, 1976.
14. Bentel, G.C. et al. *Treatment Planning and Dose Calculation*, pp. 114-116.
15. Hale, J., Davis, L.W., Bloch, P. "Portal Separation for Pairs of Parallel Opposed Portals at 2 MV and 6MV, *Am J Roentgenol* 14:172, 1972.
16. Perez, C.A. & Brady, L.W. *Principles and Practice of Radiation Oncology*, J.B. Lippincott, Philadelphia, 1987, p. 425.

Effects Of Tissue Inhomogeneity

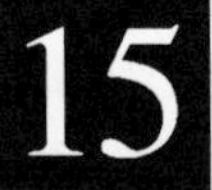

People are not homogenized internally. The fact that details of internal structure are discernable on a radiograph implies that radiation can distinguish between non-similar tissues. While this fact is a boon in diagnostic radiology, it is usually a bane in radiotherapy.

Thus far, we have considered dosimetry only in media whose properties did not vary from point to point in the fields (with the exception of our discussion of the effects of heterogeneities on electron beams). Since it is sometimes necessary to take into account the effect of tissue dissimilarities on radiation beams, we must now consider methods for doing so.

A.
Nature of the Differences

Other than differences in size and shape, there are basically only two differences between non-similar tissues such as muscle, bone, lung, fat, and air. These are electron density and effective atomic number.

Effective atomic number is important only when one is using soft radiations (orthovoltage and under), or when using very high radiation (above 10 MV). In the realm between these modes, the only important type of absorption is due to Compton effect, the probability of which does not depend on atomic number, but upon electron density. For photon energies encountered in the orthovoltage and superficial ranges, the photoelectric effect accounts for a significant portion of the absorption, and in fact becomes extremely important in superficial irradiation. The probability of the photoelectric effect depends strongly on atomic number.

For very high energy photons, a significant portion of the total absorption may be due to the process of pair production, whose probability is directly proportional to the atomic number of the absorber.

For all photon energies, the electron density is an important factor. Electron density was discussed briefly in Chapter 5, Section G. It is defined as the number of electrons per cubic centimeter of the absorber. It can be found as the product of the mass density (grams per cm^3) and the number of electrons per gram of the medium; i.e.:

$$electron\ density = \frac{electrons}{cm^3} = \frac{grams}{cm^3} \cdot \frac{electrons}{grams}$$

The number of electrons per gram of typical body tissues were listed in Chapter 5, Section G, and again here.

Table 15.1:

Medium	Density Range (gram/cm^3)	Electrons /gram
water	1.0	3.34×10^{23}
air	0.0013	3.01×10^{23}
muscle	1	3.31×10^{23}
bone	1.1 - 1.8	3.19×10^{23}
fat	0.9 - 0.95	3.37×10^{23}

The distressing aspect of Table 15.1 is the great variation in the density of bone and, to a lesser degree, fat. Some bony structures, such as the extremity bones, are dense and compact in structure, where as some, such as the sternum, are spongy and not much denser than the surrounding soft tissues. Thus, if one devises a method for determining the size and location of a bone structure (and this in itself is no mean task), there may still be a considerable uncertainty concerning its effect on a radiation beam.

B.
Nature of the Effects

Three factors are involved in causing a change in the expected dose in and near an inhomogeneity. First, the degree of attenuation of primary radiation is altered. This is the most obvious change, and the only one which may be quantitatively predicted if one has the information about electron density and effective atomic number. This change has an effect on the dose within the inhomogeneity and beyond it, but has no effect on the overlying tissue.

Secondly, there are changes due to alteration in the pattern of scattered radiation. This causes changes in dose not only to the inhomogeneity and the tissue beyond, but also to the overlying tissue, because of altered backscatter. This latter effect will be ignored in calculation, sometimes because the effect is very small, and sometimes because there currently exists no technique for dealing with the problem. One can say, however, that dose changes due to altered scattering will be more important for softer radiation, and less important for hard x-rays, since both forward and backward scattering decrease at higher initial photon energies. (Actually, scattering corresponds to the only effective absorption method at the higher energies, but it is scattering through very small angles, and behaves much like the accompanying primary radiation.)

The third alteration is in the flux distribution of the secondary electrons; i.e., a loss of electronic equilibrium at and near boundaries. We have already considered certain aspects of this; for example, an unwanted partial regaining of the tissue sparing (skin sparing) effect just after passing from a less dense medium to a dense one (refer back to Chapter 4, Section A), as in going from the lung to a solid tumor, or in passing out of the trachea. We have also discussed electron "contamination" of the skin due to the proximity of dense structures such as field shaping blocks or shadow trays. This same phenomenon occurs internally at a bone-soft tissue interface. When a radiation beam passes from bone to soft tissue, the soft tissue near the boundary receives a higher than usual dose because of an increased electron flux in the bone. Soft tissue is thus affected within a distance of up to 40 or 50 microns from the boundary (on both sides), and is much more pronounced for soft radiation. A similar phenomenon occurs when a radiation beam passes from any dense to less dense medium, such as when passing from chest wall into lung.

Alteration in electron flux is also related to the often large difference in dose between different tissues because of f-factor differences. These ideas are illustrated in Figure 15.1. Consider a layer of bone imbedded in muscle, irradiated by photons in the low orthovoltage range:

Figure 15.1

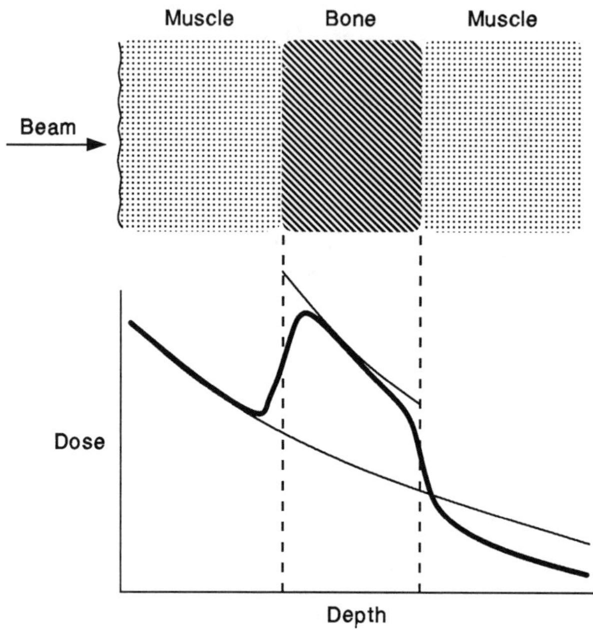

In the graph, the dashed line represents the depth dose curve as it would appear in a homogeneous muscle medium. The solid curve - the actual dose - is seen to follow the dashed curve until we are in close proximity to the first interface, where the muscle tissue dose begins increasing due to electron contamination from the bone. Within the bone, but close to the boundary, the dose is higher, but not as high as it should be based on the increased f-factor. This is because the electron flux is still partly characteristic of nearby muscle; i.e., electronic equilibrium has not yet been regained. The dose continues higher in the bone, but the falloff slope is much greater because of the greater electron density of the bone. At the second boundary, these effects appear in reverse order, and back into the muscle tissue. The depth dose curve continues with a slope characteristic of muscle, but reduced in magnitude due to extra absorption in the overlying bone.

The foregoing discussion is most pertinent to softer radiations. For cobalt-60 photons and high energy x-rays, the absorption scheme would be as shown in Figure 15.2.

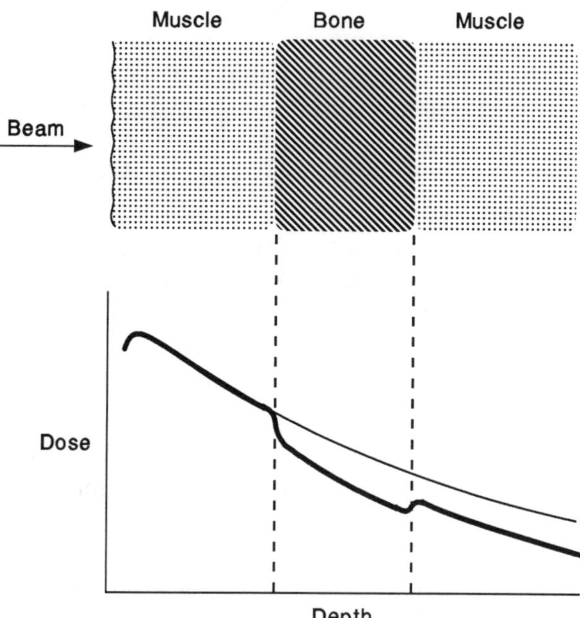

In the case of the higher energy radiation, the dose in the bone is immediately reduced because of the lower f-factor, due in turn to the lower number of electrons per gram. (Since the major absorption process is Compton effect, the higher effective atomic number of the bone has no bearing.) Again, the slope of the depth dose curve is steepened because of the higher electron density in the bone, so that the overall effect is a degradation in dose.

C.
Determining the Size and Location of an Inhomogeneity

This must be done in order to perform any sensible correction. The alternatives to this are (a) assume a homogeneous patient and make no correction, or (b) assume the patient to be "average" or "standard," and refer to a volume of illustrated cross-sectional anatomy and simply transfer such inhomogeneities as lung and large bone structures onto the patient's contour according to the sizes and locations illustrated. It is questionable whether this procedure is superior to complete avoidance of the problem by assuming a homogeneous patient. Not many cancer patients are average or standard internally. A lung may be largely filled with neoplasm or fluid and thus may be closer in electron density to muscle tissue than to normal lung tissue; or the patient may have emphysema, in which case the electron density would be that of air. A bony structure may be eroded by cancer to the point where bone may not even exist as such at the locations indicated in an anatomy text.

The most obvious method of determining size and location of internal structures is by the use of tomography, usually computed tomography (CT). One must use caution in interpreting the images in either case; use these techniques to determine size and shape only. Avoid making assumptions about the relative densities of the differing internal structures based on contrasts on the tomographs; these were seen by diagnostic x-rays, which interact with the tissues by different processes than do the therapeutic rays. With careful calibration, however, a treatment planning system can use CT numbers to correct for inhomogeneities. Computerized tomography plays a great role in accurate positioning of even many very small inhomogeneities.

Other methods which may give some information regarding the sizes and locations of internal structures are simple **orthogonal radiographs** and **ultrasound**. Both are rather restricted in what they can tell you. Orthogonal radiographs are radiographs made with central rays at right angles to each other and a common isocenter; as such they display images on a three-dimensional linear (cartesian) coordinate system. With this one can usually determine thicknesses mathematically, but it is difficult if not impossible, to place the exact location of curved boundaries. One must also be careful to take into account differing degrees of magnification on the two views, as well as varying magnification from point to point on the same view.

Ultrasound is usually even more restricted in that the very inhomogeneities one seeks act as highly effective barriers to the passage of ultrasound waves. The reflection coefficients at a soft tissue-bone interface or a muscle-lung interface are very high, so that nearly all of the sound is reflected at the first boundary, leaving very little for penetration to the interior of the inhomogeneity.[1] This is a highly useful technique for determining the size and location of that first boundary, which in some cases is all you need to know. For example, in determining the thickness of the chest wall preparatory to tangential chest treatment, you need not know what underlies this, since your aim is to avoid it.

D.

Determining the Absorption Properties of Internal Structures

The most straightforward way to accomplish this is to use a beam of the same radiation to be used in therapy.

Suppose one mounts a radiation detector on the beamstopper of a treatment unit, so that it is always a fixed distance from the source, and always coaxial with the central ray. Input to the sensitive volume of the detector is collimated through lead, the collimator holes directed toward the source, so that only primary radiation (no scatter) is detected. Such a device is called a **focusing transit dosimeter**.

Now one interposes phantoms of various water or water equivalent thicknesses, and measures the attenuation of the primary radiation as a function of thickness. This is kept as a reference table.

Now a patient is positioned in the beam. During an exposure, a measurement is made using the transit dosimeter. One can compare this reading with the reference table of water attenuation values, and make a statement such as, "This patient is equivalent to 13 cm of water."

Now this figure is coupled with a knowledge of the actual thickness of the patient, along with a knowledge of the size and location of an internal inhomogeneity (obtained from tomography, etc.) in order to determine dose at various points along the central ray.

Example 15.1:

>A patient is known to have an internal inhomogeneity of the size and location illustrated in Figure 15.3. (The structure is bone, but we really do not require this knowledge.)

Figure 15.3

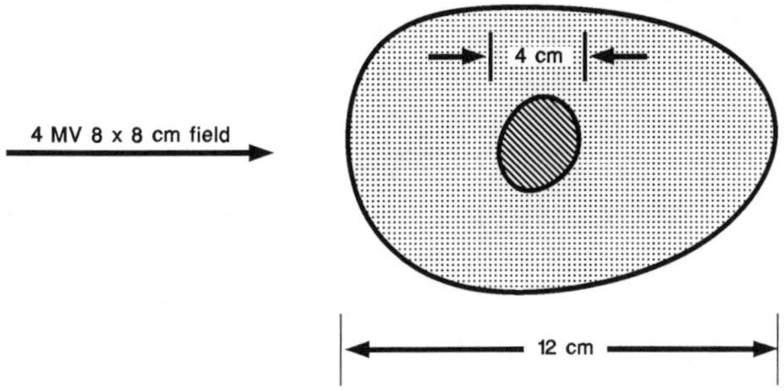

A transit dosimeter reading through the patient is compared to a table of water transmission value for the same machine, and it is determined that, through the central ray, the patient appears to be equivalent to 14.4 cm of water. The patient is known to be 12 cm thick through this ray, and has only the one inhomogeneity; the rest is assumed to be water equivalent.

From this, we can say that the inhomogeneity has an electron density 1.6 times that of water. This is so because of the 14.4 cm of water equivalent thickness, 8 cm is known to be muscle, which we are assuming to be water equivalent. The other 6.4 cm is accounted for by the 4 cm inhomogeneity, and $6.4/4.0 = 1.6$. From this point we could determine the dose at various points along this ray in a number of ways.

The assumption made here is that the separate structures are themselves homogeneous; i.e., the bone does not vary in electron density from point to point, and the tissue surrounding it is also of uniform properties. This will not necessarily be the case, but is generally the best we can do. If the point of interest lies within the inhomogeneity, the invalidity of this assumption will result in a small error; if, however, our point of interest lies after the inhomogeneity, it does not matter greatly if the properties within the inhomogeneity are uniform.

Short of actually measuring the attenuating properties of an inhomogeneity, one can approximate them from a knowledge of the average properties of that kind of tissue. For example, lung tissue has an average electron density about 0.3 times that of muscle. The electron density of bone can be anywhere from 1.1 to 1.8 times that of muscle, depending on how "spongy" it is. Bone in the extremities (e.g., femur) is generally compact and dense, whereas bone in the sternum is relatively lightweight. Obviously, it is better to be able to measure the properties.

E.
Making the Corrections

We assume now that by some hook, crook, or mystical insight we know the thickness of the inhomogeneity, its location within the cross-section, and its equivalent muscle thickness, which is equal to its actual thickness times a ratio of its electron density to the electron density of muscle. We also have sufficient information available to enable us to calculate what the dose would be in the absence of the inhomogeneity. This in fact is our first step - we calculate the dose at points of interest assuming that the inhomogeneity is not different from muscle. Our job is then to apply a correction factor to these calculated doses. The first method, the **tissue-air ratio method,** involves using a ratio of TAR's (or TMR's or TPR's). Refer to Figure 15.4.

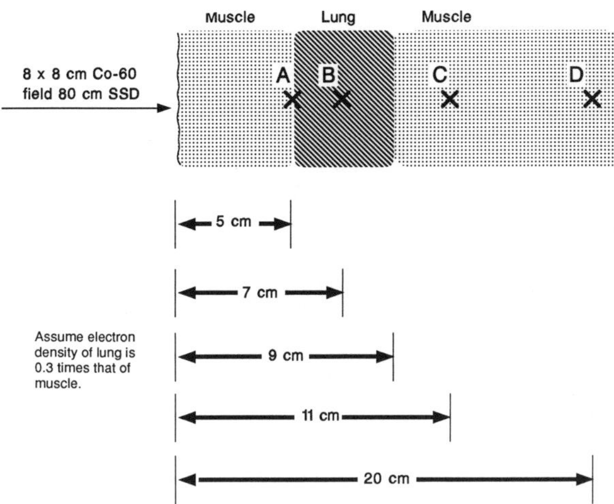

A layer of low density medium 4 cm thick is sandwiched between layers of muscle. The layer begins 5 cm below the surface. Points A, B, C, and D lie on the central ray of an 8 x 8 cm cobalt-60 field whose SSD is 80 cm.

First, we find the depth dose fractions to points A, B, C, and D as if there were no inhomogeneity. These are 0.780, 0.682, 0.512, and 0.261 respectively, from the depth dose table for a cobalt-60 unit.

Now we calculate the effective thickness of tissue overlying each point. (This is not the same as an effective depth, because of inverse square law considerations.) For point A, this is still 5 cm, since no lung overlies this point. Thus the depth dose fraction will remain 0.780. In this, we are neglecting the effect of loss of backscatter due to the presence of lung. The actual dose to point A will be slightly less than our estimate.

Point B lies at the midpoint of the layer of lung. The muscle equivalent thickness of 2 cm of lung having a relative electron density of 0.3 is 0.3 x 2 cm = 0.6 cm; this, along with the 5 cm of muscle tissue, gives an equivalent muscle thickness of 5.6 cm.

Point C lies below a total of 5 cm + 2 cm = 7 cm of muscle, and 4 cm of lung, having an equivalent muscle thickness of 4 x 0.3 cm = 1.2 cm, for a total effective muscle thickness of 8.2 cm; Point D, 5 cm + 1.2 cm + 11 cm = 17.2 cm.

We now obtain for each point a ratio of TAR's under two conditions: TAR for depth corresponding to effective muscle thickness, and TAR for actual depth. We use TAR's instead of ddf's because we are considering the same point under two absorption conditions, rather than two points at different distances from the source. Ideally, the TAR's should correspond to field sizes as measured at the depth of interest and not the field size at the surface; however, while TAR varies noticeably with field size, the variation of such ratios of TAR's varies only slightly. Consider the TAR ratio at 8 cm and 10 cm depths for a field size of 8 x 8 cm, for example, and the same sort of ratio for a field size of 12 x 12 cm:

$$\frac{\text{TAR}\left(8 \times 8 \text{ cm, } 8 \text{ cm}\right)}{\text{TAR}\left(8 \times 8 \text{ cm, } 10 \text{ cm}\right)} = \frac{0.717}{0.653} = 1.098$$

$$\frac{\text{TAR}\left(12 \times 12 \text{ cm, } 8 \text{ cm}\right)}{\text{TAR}\left(12 \times 12 \text{ cm, } 10 \text{ cm}\right)} = \frac{0.750}{0.683} = 1.098$$

thus a minimal error results if we consider only the field size at the normalization depth. The ratios are:

$$\text{for point } B, \frac{TAR\ (5.6)}{TAR\ (7.0} = \frac{0.873}{0.819} = 1.066$$

$$\text{for point } C, \frac{TAR\ (8.2)}{TAR\ (11.0)} = \frac{0.778}{0.684} = 1.137$$

$$\text{for point } D, \frac{TAR\ (17.2)}{TAR\ (20.0)} = \frac{0.502}{0.436} = 1.151$$

As a first approximation, we could apply these as multiplicative correction factors to the respective ddf's, TAR and TMR. For SAD planning, this is equivalent to using effective thickness, rather than actual depth, to determine TARs or TMRs.

The second method, the **effective attention method**, is a refinement of the TAR method. It includes a correction for the fact that the buildup of dose due to scattered photons in and below the inhomogeneity does not occur totally for several centimeters, just as this is true within normal muscle tissue. For this reason, the figures above must usually be amended by a position correction factor, which is a function of how far the point in question lies below the inhomogeneity. This position correction factor is actually a function of field size, photon energy size of the inhomogenous structure, and distance from it to the point of interest. In general, the position correction factor will be closer to unity for higher energy radiations, larger field sizes, smaller heterogeneities, and greater distance between the inhomogeneity and the field point. However, as is usually the case when many variables are involved, average values are recommended for use. The values in Table 15.2 are taken from ICRU Report 24, and were determined experimentally and averaged for cobalt-60 and 4MV x-rays.[1]

Table 15.2

cm from heterogeneity to field point	0	2	5	>10
position correction factor	0.92	0.95	0.97	1.0

In our example, point B would have a position correction factor of 0.92, since it is within the inhomogeneity; point C would have a correction of 0.95; and point D would have a correction of 1.0 (i.e., no position correction).

Thus, the ddf's would be corrected as follows:

Point	ddf with no heterogeneity	TAR ratio correction	Position correction	Corrected ddf
A	0.780	1.00	1.00	0.780
B	0.682	1.066	0.92	0.669
C	0.512	1.137	0.95	0.553
D	0.261	1.151	1.00	0.300

Observe that the dose to point B, the point within the inhomogeneity, appears to have been reduced even though some of the attenuating material above it is of lower electron density. This may or may not be true. Corrections to dose for points within a inhomogeneity are highly suspect and are difficult to assess, because of the loss of electronic equilibrium and rebuilding of the photon scatter pattern.

In addition, there is a third method known as the **power law tissue-air ratio method**, the **Butho-Young-Gaylord method**, or simply the **power law method**.[2,3,4,5,6] This method produces a more accurate result, but it involves more complex calculations. The interested reader should refer to the references. However, the most recently developed method used to correct for tissue inhomogeneity, the **equivalent TAR method**, uses computer tomography.[7] This may be the most accurate method for correcting tissue inhomogeneity for dose calculation.

F.
Making Corrections to Isodose Distributions by Hand

For this, a fourth method, which is a modification of the isodose shift method, may be used to correct for internal inhomogeneities. That is, after the isodose shift corrections have been made to the isodose curves because of air gap at the surface, they are applied again to compensate for heterogeneities if they overlie the isodose lines. For this, a shift fraction is used which is characteristic of the type of inhomogeneity. (By shift fraction is meant the distance that the isodose line is shifted along the diverging ray pattern, divided by the thickness of the inhomogeneity measured along the ray.)

The following shift fractions are recommended in ICRU report 24, for cobalt-60 and 4MV radiations.[8] Smaller shifts would be valid for higher energy radiations.

Nature of Inhomogeneity	Shift Fraction
air cavity	-0.6
lung tissue	-0.4
hard bone	+0.5
spongy bone	+0.25

A minus shift fraction means the shift should be away from the skin, and a positive shift would be made toward the skin.

In this method, in order to correct for an inhomogeneity, the isodose lines are shifted by an amount equal to the shift fraction times the thickness of inhomogeneity as measured along a line parallel to the axis of the central ray and passing through the point at which dose is calculated.

Thus, if one of the lines in the diverging ray pattern passes through 5 cm of lung tissue, the isodose lines below this lung should be shifted along that ray a distance of 5 cm x (-0.4) = -2.0 cm, (2 cm away from the surface).

References

1. International Commission on Radiation Units. *Determination of Absorbed Dose in a Patient Irradiated by Beams of X or Gamma Rays in Radiotherapy Procedures*, Report #24, International Commission on Radiation Units and Measurements, Washington, D.C., 1976, p. 23.
2. Butho, H.F. "Lung Corrections in Cobalt-60 Beam Therapy," *J Canad Assn Radio* 15,79, 1964.
3. Young, M.E.J. and Gaylord, J.D. "Experimental Tests of Corrections for Tissue Inhomogeneities in Radiotherapy," *Br J Radiol* 43, 349, 1970.
4. Johns & Cunningham, *The Physics of Radiology*, 4th Edition, C.C. Thomas, Springfield, 1983, p. 392-393.
5. Khan, F. *The Physics of Radiation Therapy*, Williams & Wilkins, 1984, p. 256.
6. Sonntag, M.R. & Cunningham, J.R. "Corrections to Absorbed Dose Calculations for Tissue Inhomogeneities, " *Med Phys* 4: 431, 1977.
7. Sonntag, M.R. & Cunningham, J.R. "The Equivalent Tissue-Air Ratio Method for Making Absorbed Dose Culculations in Heterogeneous Medium," *Radiology*, 129:787-794, 1978.
8. ICRU Report #24, p. 23.

Tissue Compensation

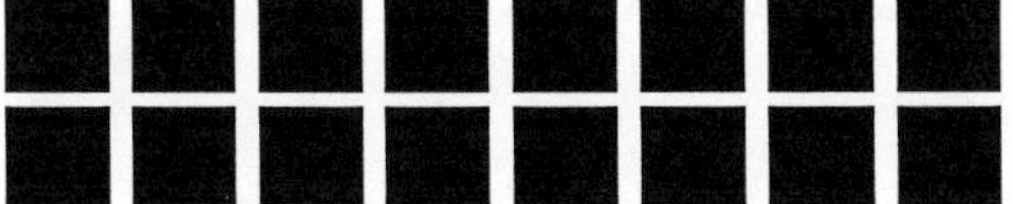

16

A. An Example Illustrating the Need for a Compensation
B. Compensation by Blocking and Boosting
C. Compensation Using Wedges
D. Custom Made Compensators

Compensators are frequently called compensating filters, but as in the case of beam flattening "filters," this is playing fast and loose with the term filter, which should mean a device for selectively absorbing photons of differing energies.

There are many situations which lead to an inhomogeneous dose throughout a target volume. For example, the presence of tissue inhomogeneity, sloping skin surface, and most often, differing patient thickness over the range of the target volume.

A compensator is a device used to compensate for these factors, and thus regain homogeneity within the target volume. However, there are instances when a compensator might be used to do the opposite; i.e., to create a dose inhomogeneity of a controlled nature.

The compensator is most often a physical device made of some material which may be either roughly tissue equivalent or may be of metal, such as aluminum, brass, or lead. However, the "compensator" may not be a physically present device at all; for example, it may consist of the simple expedient of varying the field sizes during the overall treatment schedule.

A.
An Example Illustrating the Need for a Compensator

Descriptions of the construction and use of compensators are best done by example. We shall therefore frequently use the following example in this section.

Figure 16.1

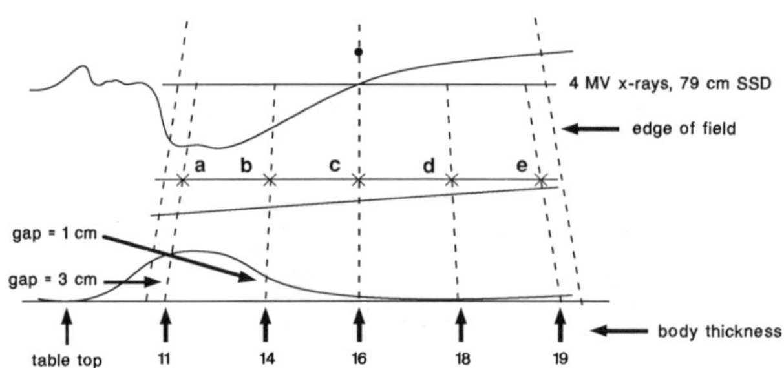

A 16 x 16 cm field of 4 MV x-rays at 79 cm SSD (measured to central ray) is incident on a sloping chest and neck. In practice, this would most probably be one of an opposing pair, but we shall consider only the anterior field, since compensation for the other field would utilize the same technique. In fact, it is possible to do all needed compensation from one side only for simplicity, but we shall not do this in our example.

Figure 16.2 shows an isodose summation in the above case, when no compensation is used.

Figure 16.2

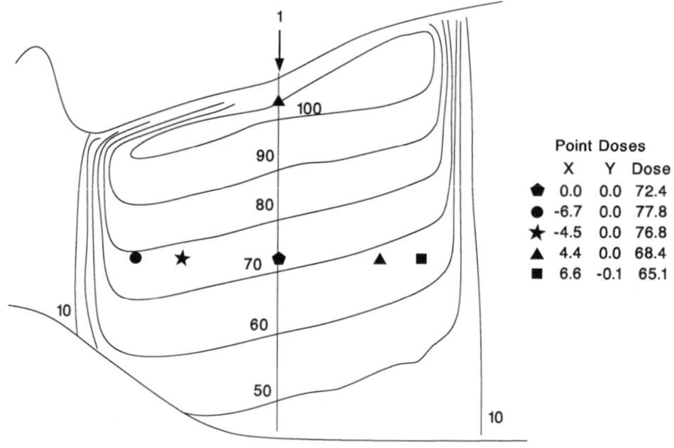

At midline, the dose range is from 61.7% to 78% of maximum dose; a total variation of 18% of the dose at point C. This is unacceptable. (Note: We are not considering tissues within 1 cm of the field edge. It would be foolish to attempt to compensate for penumbra.)

B.

Compensation by Blocking and Boosting

Suppose we are attempting to give 30 Gy in 15 fractions from this field to the midline of the patient with an allowable range of ±3%. Without compensation, in order for the dose at point C to be 30 Gy, the dose at point A will be 32.2 Gy (+7.3%, i.e., 7.3% more than the dose at point C); at point B it will be 31.8 Gy (+6%); at point D it will be 28.3 Gy (-5.5%); and at point E it will be 27 Gy (-10.1%).

We could remedy this by reducing the dose at points A and B, and boosting the dose at points D and E. For example, if we were to insert a block over the upper 1/3 of the field during one of the 15 fractions, the dose to points A and B would be reduced by approximately [0.95 x (1/15)], or 6.3%. (The 0.95 assumes a 5% block transmission, and this ignores lateral scattering from the remaining portion of the field.) Thus, the overall dose to point A would be (1 - 0.063) x 32.2 Gy = 30.2 Gy (+0.7); the dose at point B would become (1 - 0.063) x 31.8 Gy = 29.8 Gy (-0.7%).

Suppose now we align a separate small boost field over the lower 1/4 of the field. We shall deliver 2.5 Gy to midline from this field in order to bring the dose to point E to a total of 29.5 Gy (-1.6%). The dose to point D would then be approximately 28.3 Gy + 2.5 Gy = 30.8 Gy (+2.7%).

Figure 16.3 shows the result of this compensation by boosting and blocking. Some point doses are slightly different from what we calculated above, since the computer which generated the iso-dose curves did not make as many approximations.

Figure 16.3

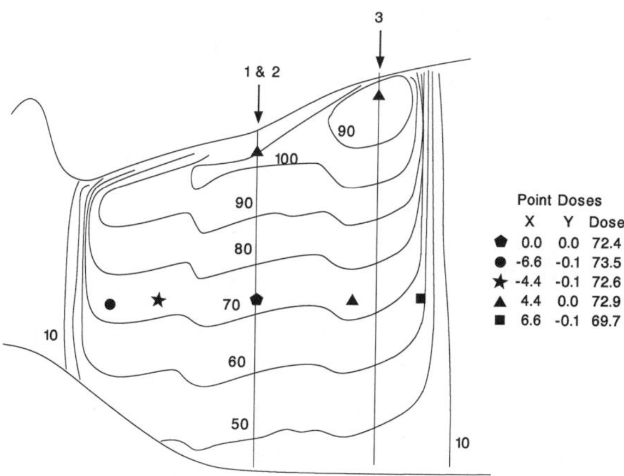

While this method is universally applicable, it has a few serious drawbacks. First, it obviously complicates the set-up procedure for both simulation and set-up. This always increases the chance for error, as well as increasing the general level of confusion. If the above case involved opposing fields, there would be eight sets of set-up involved.

Secondly, using such a technique subjects different portions of the target volume to different time-dose-fractionation schedules. While it is difficult to quantitatively assess the degree of difference in biological response, it can be stated with confidence that there will be some difference.

C.
Compensation Using Wedges

We have already encountered an example of this; treatment of the larynx with opposing lateral fields as discussed in Chapter 11, Section F.

Compensation is possible by this means only if the surface irregularities and thickness differences are uniform in extent; e.g., treatment through a body section which continuously thins across the field, rather than thinning and rethickening. Figure 16.4 shows this technique applied to our test case of the sloping chest.

Figure 16.4

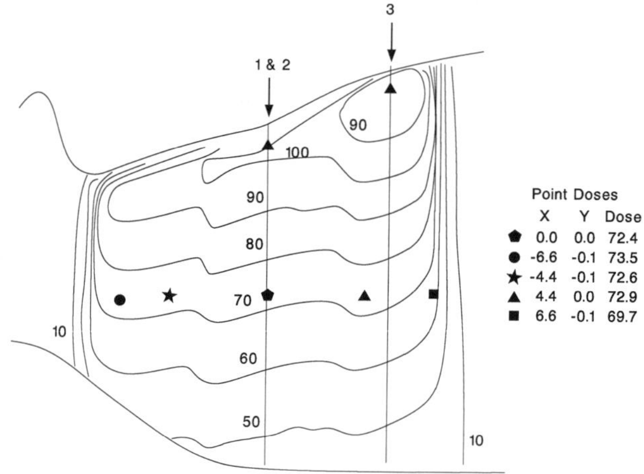

Observe that this is a combination of an open field and a 30° wedged field (wedge factor of 0.712) respective weights 60:40, simulating a single field of weight 100.

An obvious limitation to this technique, in addition to the one mentioned above, is that most wedges permit field lengths up to only 16 cm or so. Thus medium large and large fields cannot be compensated totally in this manner.

D.
Custom Made Compensators

Since the primary reason for using some form of compensation is to counteract differences in patient thickness (or in the case of a single field, differences in depth to a line or plane of interest), it would seem that the most straightforward approach would be to fill in the irregularities with some tissue-like phantom material (bolus) so that the depths or thicknesses are uniform, as in Figure 16.5.

Figure 16.5

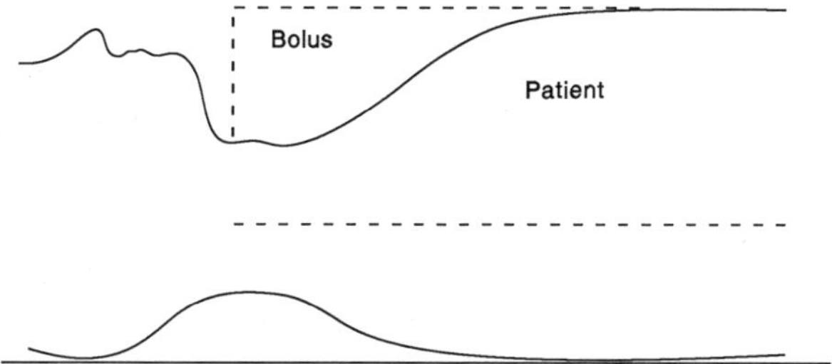

This, however, would cause an unacceptable skin dose to occur in most cases. Thus an approach frequently taken is to displace the bolus upward away from the skin (to a shadow tray, for example) demagnifying it, since it will be closer to the source, as in Figure 16.6.

Figure 16.6

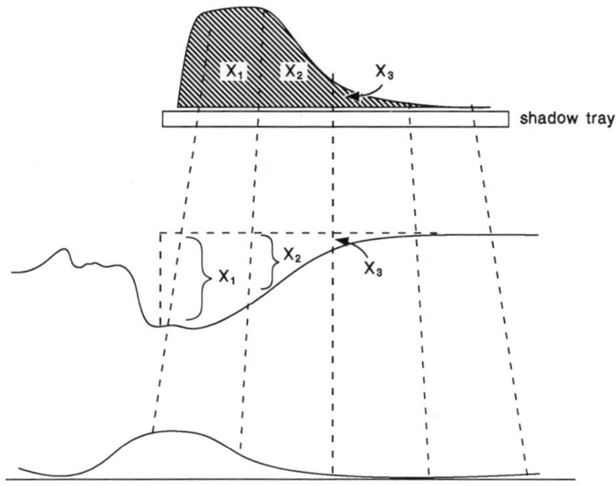

By **demagnifying** is meant the compression of the lateral dimension only (the dimensions perpendicular to the central ray). The thickness through each diverging ray would be left unchanged. This demagnification is most simply done by drawing the patient section and shadow tray in proper geometric relations and overlaying a diverging ray pattern. Then one simply transposes the correct thickness upward along each shadow tray until a profile can be drawn of the demagnified "bolus". This assumes that the bolus consists of tissue equivalent material. If this is not so, the thicknesses would also be scaled upward or downward in accordance with their departure from tissue equivalence. For example, if the compensator is to be of brass with an electron density eight times that of tissue, the thicknesses would be scaled down to one-eighth, assuming the radiation is from cobalt or some unit of higher energy. For lower energy radiations, using a higher atomic number would be unwise because of differences in the absorption processes (Compton vs. photoelectric effects). In any case, the procedure of separating the bolus from the skin is not required for these energies, since there is no noticeable skin sparing effect to lose by using a conventional bolus.

There are two major faults in this procedure. First, by doing this, one is attempting to restore the isodose distribution to the appearance it has upon entering perpendicularly into a flat surfaced phantom. This is not necessarily desirable, since one would still have either falloff or "horns" toward the edge of the field. If one takes the trouble to build a compensator, why not attempt to do away with these usually undesirable characteristics?

Secondly, there is the assumption that separating the bolus from the skin causes no change in the required thickness. This is not so, since the scattered photon flux will be altered. It was pointed out in an earlier section that the scattered photon dose describes a buildup curve just as the secondary electrons do, except on a much larger scale. The peak dose due to scattered photons will occur at some depth in the range from six to fifteen centimeters depending on field size and photon energy. If the bolus is in contact with the skin, this buildup need occur only once; however, when the bolus is separated from the skin the scatter buildup is partially lost (just as electron buildup is), and must be recovered. Since scattered photons account for a non-negligable portion of the dose, this may result in an error of several percent.

To illustrate the magnitude of this error, consider Table 16.1. This presents the results of measurements performed in a muscle equivalent (polystyrene) phantom irradiated by a cobalt-60 beam and 10 MV x-ray beam. The column labelled "depth" refers to depth in a simulated patient, not including a 4 cm layer of "compensator" (of the same material). Thus, for a nominal depth of 5 cm, the radiation has actually passed through 9 cm of polystyrene. Dose was measured first with the 4 cm compensator directly on the "skin", then separated from the skin by the shadow tray height (15 - 20 cm). The column labelled "dose ratio" gives the ratio of the second measurement to the first, and the next column lists the percent error. In each case, the field size at the surface was 15 x 15 cm, and the phantom was semi-infinite.

Table 16.1:

Treatment Unit	Depth	Dose Ratio	% Error
Cobalt-60	1	0.869	13.1
	5	0.914	9.6
	10	0.943	5.7
Clinac 18	2	0.948	5.2
	5	0.961	3.9
	10	0.920	8.0

Note that in each case the error is unacceptable. The obvious conclusion is that this technique should not be used.

For an approximate method of designing compensators which gives acceptably close results, refer back to our example patient of Figure 16.2.

Consider the rays leading to the points A and E, equidistant from the central ray. The tissue thickness above point A is 6.3 cm and for point E is 10.7 cm. The difference between them is 4.4 cm. Thus, if one took the simple approach just discussed, he would place a compensator on the shadow tray whose thickness along the ray A is 4.8 cm, the purpose of this being to reduce the ddf at point A from 0.750 to 0.639, thus making it equal to the ddf at point E. As we have just seen, this would result in an underdose at the "compensated" point A, an error of approximately four or five percent.

Instead, we first determine the degree of reduction necessary at point A in order to give it the same ddf as point E. This is 0.639/0.750 = 0.852. Next we go to a TMR table for this radiation quality and seek out the TMR for this field size, at 10.7 cm depth (point E), obtaining a value of 0.749. Now we ask what additional thickness (beyond 10.7 cm) is required to give us a reduction to 0.852 of this value; i.e., at what depth does the TMR = 0.852 x 0.749 = 0.638? From the TMR table, we see that this depth is 14.6 cm. Thus, an additional 3.9 cm gives the required reduction (14.6 cm - 10.7 cm).

Thus, this method tells· us to use 5 mm less compensator thickness than does the previous method. This corresponds to a dose difference of about 2.5%, which is approximately the error resulting from the simplified method of using a compensator thickness equal to the tissue thickness difference.

You may now ask why we selected a starting depth of 10.7 cm, rather than the depth of maximum dose (d_{max}). The answer is that at 10.7 cm, the scattered radiation has effectively reached its maximum buildup, for all but very large fields. Note that if we had chosen the additional thickness beyond d_{max} to achieve a dose reduction to 0.852, we would have required about 7 cm.

If this same procedure is repeated for several points, a cross-sectional profile of the compensator may be deduced. Then the compensator is demagnified as before and placed on the shadow tray.

Some Constants and Conversion Factors

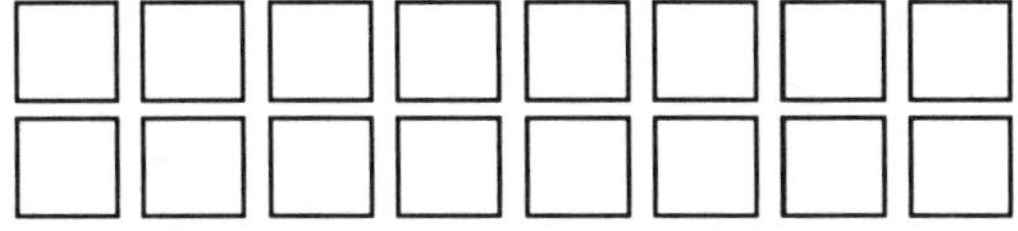 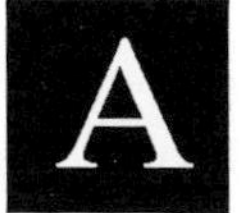

Electron volt	$1 \text{ eV} = 1.60 \times 10^{-19} \text{ J}$
Joule	$1 \text{ J} = 1 \text{ kg m}^2/\text{s}^2 = 10^7 \text{ erg}$
Roentgen	$1 \text{ R} = 2.58 \times 10^{-4}$ c/kg air $= 3.336 \times 10^{-10}$ c/cm^3 air at STP [Standard Temperature (0° C) and Atmospheric Pressure (760 mm Hg)]
Gray	$1 \text{ Gy} = 1 \text{ J/kg}$
Rad	$1 \text{ Rad} = 1 \text{ cGy} = 0.01 \text{ Gy} = 100 \text{ erg/g}$
Becquerel	$1 \text{ Bq} = 1.0 \text{ dps} = 2.7 \times 10^{-11} \text{ Ci}$
Curie*	$1 \text{ Ci} = 3.7 \times 10^{10} \text{ dps} = 3.7 \times 10^{10} \text{ Bq}$
Micron	10^{-6} m
Electron: rest mass charge (-e)	$m_e = 9.11 \times 10^{-31} \text{ kg}$ $1e = 1.6 \times 10^{-19} \text{ C}$
Positron: rest mass charge (+e)	$m_{positron} = 9.11 \times 10^{-31} \text{ kg}$ $1e = 1.6 \times 10^{-19} \text{ C}$

---

* 1 Curie is based on the rate of decay of 1 gram of radium which is equal to 3.7×10^{10} disintegration per second (dps). Recent measurement found this value to be 3.61×10^{10} dps per gram of radium. However, the original definition of Curie remains the same.

Neutron:
rest mass $m_n = 1.675 \times 10^{-27}$ kg
charge (0)   0

Proton:
rest mass $m_p = 1.673 \times 10^{-27}$ kg
charge (+e) $1e = 1.6 \times 10^{-19}$ C

Speed of light
in free space $c = 3.0 \times 10^8$ m/s $= 1.86 \times 10^5$ mi/s

1 kilgram   1 kg = 1000 grams (g)

1 meter   1 m = 100 cm = 3.28 ft = 39.4 in

1 kilometer   1 km = 1000 m = 0.621 mi

1 foot   1 ft = 12 in = 0.305 m = 30.5 cm

1 mile   1 mi = 5280 ft = 1.61 km

Superficial X-Ray Unit

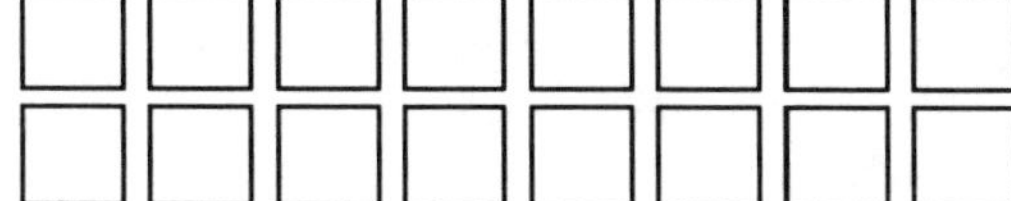 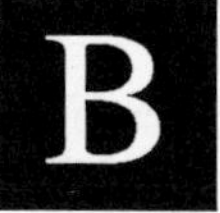

Superficial X-Ray Unit
Universal X-Ray, Tube Serial #0331

Indicated kVP	Indicated mA	Added Filter	HVL (mm AL)	Target Skin dist.	Cone Diameter	cGy/min (in air)	cGy/* min
90	5	0	.4	13.5 cm	2 cm	711	663
90	5	0	.4	13.5 cm	5 cm	766	756
90	5	0	.4	31.3 cm	16.5 cm	137	145
90	5	.5mm AL	1.1	13.5 cm	2 cm	322	305
90	5	.5mm AL	1.1	13.4 cm	5 cm	356	373
90	5	.5mm AL	1.1	31.3 cm	16.5 cm	64	72
90	5	1.0mm AL	1.7	13.5 cm	2 cm	217	208
90	5	1.0mm AL	1.7	13.5 cm	5 cm	246	258
90	5	1.0mm AL	1.7	31.3 cm	16.5 cm	44	51

*cGy per minute data <u>include</u> backscatter factors

Useful Data:

HVL (mm AL)	Effective Photon Energy	cGy/R (f-factor)
0.4	17 kev	0.905
1.1	24 kev	0.903
1.7	28 kev	0.904

Backscatter Factors

Field Diameter (cm)

HVL (mm AL)	0	1	2	3	4	5
0.4	1.00	1.01	1.03	1.06	1.08	109
1.1	1.00	1.02	1.05	1.09	1.12	1.14
1.7	1.00	1.02	1.06	1.10	1.12	1.16

Field Diameter (cm)

VL nm AL)	0	2	4	6	8	10	12	14	16	18
0.4	1.00	1.03	1.08	1.11	1.13	1.14	1.15	1.16	1.17	1.17
1.1	1.00	1.05	1.12	1.16	1.18	1.20	1.22	1.23	1.24	1.25
1.7	1.00	1.06	1.12	1.18	1.20	1.23	1.25	1.26	1.27	1.28

Instruments Used:
Victoreen Model 500, Serial #303
Model #500-14 Chamber, Serial #107
Readings corrected for tempurature
and pressure.

cGy per minute versus field size (Using 5 cm cone with lead cutouts)
Effective circle diameter (cm)

HVL (mm AL)	1	1.5	2	3	4	5
0.4	700	707	714	735	749	756
1.1	328	331	338	350	360	373
1.7	227	231	236	245	249	258

cGy per minute vesus field size (Using 16.5 cm cone with lead cutouts)
Effective circle diameter (cm)

HVL (mm AL)	5	6	8	10	12	14	16	18
0.4	135	136	140	141	143	144	145	145
1.1	65.9	67.0	68.2	69.4	70.5	71.1	71.1	72.2
1.7	46.1	46.9	47.7	48.9	49.7	50.1	50.5	50.9

Depth Dose Fractions
HVL = 0.4 mm AL, TSD = 13.5 cm, 5 cm cone

Field Diameter (cm)

Depth (cm)	0	1	2	3	4	5
0	1.00	1.00	1.00	1.00	1.00	1.00
.1	.84	.85	.85	.86	.86	.86
.2	.74	.75	.75	.76	.76	.76
.3	.65	.66	.66	.67	.67	.67
.4	.58	.59	.59	.60	.60	.60
.5	.53	.54	.54	.55	.55	.55
.7	.44	.45	.45	.46	.46	.46
1.0	.34	.35	.35	.36	.36	.36
1.5	.23	.24	.24	.25	.25	.25
2.0	.15	.16	.16	.17	.17	.17
3.0	.07	.08	.08	.09	.09	.09

Depth Dose Fractions
HVL = 0.4 mm AL, TSD = 31.3 cm, 5 cm cone

Field Diameter (cm)

Depth (cm)	0	2	4	6	8	10 - 18
0	1.00	1.00	1.00	1.00	1.00	1.00
.1	.85	.86	.86	.86	.86	.87
.2	.77	.78	.78	.78	.78	.79
.3	.69	.70	.70	.70	.70	.71
.4	.62	.63	.63	.63	.63	.64
.5	.56	.57	.57	.57	.57	.58
.7	.47	.48	.48	.48	.48	.49
1.0	.36	.36	.37	.37	.37	.38
1.5	.25	.25	.26	.26	.26	.27
2.0	.18	1.8	.19	.19	.19	.20
3.0	.08	.09	.10	.10	.10	.11

Depth Dose Fractions
HVL = 1.1 mm AL, TSD = 13.5 cm, 5 cm cone

Field Diameter (cm)

Depth (cm)	0.0	1.0	2.0	3.0	4.0	5.0
0.0	1.000	1.000	1.000	1.000	1.000	1.000
.1	.928	.938	.947	.953	.955	.958
.2	.855	.877	.895	.905	.911	.915
.3	.784	.815	.842	.858	.866	.873
.4	.712	.754	.790	.811	.822	.831
.5	.640	.693	.738	.764	.778	.790
.7	.559	.615	.664	.694	.711	.722
1.0	.438	.499	.555	.590	.611	.622
2.0	.236	.284	.328	.359	.379	.391
3.0	.140	.170	.200	.224	.242	.252
4.0	.088	.108	.127	.143	.156	.167
5.0	.057	.070	.083	.095	.105	.113
6.0	.037	.046	.055	.064	.071	.077
7.0	.025	.031	.037	.044	.049	.054
8.0	.016	.021	.026	.031	.035	.039
9.0	.011	.014	.018	.021	.025	.028

Depth Dose Fractions
HVL = 1.7 mm AL, TSD = 13.5 cm, 5 cm cone

Field Diameter (cm)

Depth (cm)	0.0	1.0	2.0	3.0	4.0	5.0
0.0	1.000	1.000	1.000	1.000	1.000	1.000
.1	.937	.946	.954	.959	.962	.964
.2	.875	.892	.907	.918	.924	.929
.3	.812	.838	.861	.877	.887	.894
.4	.750	.784	.815	.837	.849	.859
.5	.688	.730	.769	.796	.812	.823
.7	.611	.658	.702	.734	.753	.765
1.0	.496	.550	.602	.641	.665	.679
2.0	.287	.335	.381	.417	.443	.460
3.0	.180	.213	.246	.278	.300	.312
4.0	.116	.141	.165	.185	.200	.213
5.0	.078	.095	.112	.127	.139	.150
6.0	.053	.065	.078	.089	.099	.108
7.0	.036	.045	.054	.063	.071	.079
8.0	.025	.032	.039	.045	.052	.058
9.0	.017	.023	.028	.033	.038	.044

Depth Dose Fractions
HVL = 1.1 mm AL, TSD = 31.3 cm, long metal cone

Field Diameter (cm)

Depth (cm)	0.0	2.0	4.0	6.0	8.0	10.0	14.0	16.0	18.0
0.0	1.000	1.000	1.000	1.000	1.000	1.000	1.000	1.000	1.000
.1	.933	.953	.961	.963	.965	.965	.967	.968	.968
.2	.867	.905	.921	.927	.929	.930	.934	.936	.937
.3	.800	.858	.882	.890	.894	.896	.901	.904	.905
.4	.733	.810	.842	.853	.859	.861	.868	.871	.874
.5	.666	.763	.803	.816	.823	.826	.834	.839	.842
.7	.589	.695	.740	.755	.764	.767	.777	.782	.785
1.0	.474	.593	.646	.663	.674	.679	.690	.696	.699
2.0	.273	.372	.422	.442	.454	.458	.472	.479	.483
3.0	.173	.237	.280	.300	.312	.319	.331	.336	.343
4.0	.115	.159	.190	.209	.221	.226	.238	.243	.246
5.0	.080	.106	.132	.147	.158	.163	.175	.181	.184
6.0	.055	.075	.092	.106	.116	.121	.130	.134	.137
7.0	.038	.052	.066	.077	.086	.090	.098	.103	.106
8.0	.027	.037	.047	.057	.065	.068	.076	.080	.084
9.0	.019	.027	.035	.042	.048	.051	.057	.059	.062

Depth Dose Fractions
HVL = 1.7 mm AL, TSD = 31.3 cm, long metal cone

Field Diameter (cm)

Depth (cm)	0.0	2.0	4.0	6.0	8.0	10.0	12.0	14.0	16.0	18.0
0.0	1.000	1.000	1.000	1.000	1.000	1.000	1.000	1.000	1.000	1.000
.1	.943	.960	.968	.971	.973	.974	.975	.976	.977	.978
.2	.887	.919	.936	.943	.947	.948	.950	.953	.955	.956
.3	.830	.879	.904	.914	.920	.923	.926	.929	.932	.934
.4	.773	.838	.872	.886	.893	.897	.901	.905	.910	.912
.5	.716	.798	.840	.857	.867	.871	.876	.882	.887	.890
.7	.644	.738	.787	.807	.820	.826	.833	.838	.844	.847
1.0	.536	.647	.708	.733	.750	.759	.767	.774	.780	.783
2.0	.333	.438	.503	.534	.552	.560	.568	.575	.582	.587
3.0	.222	.300	.355	.385	.405	.415	.426	.435	.444	.451
4.0	.154	.211	.252	.280	.297	.310	.322	.331	.340	.345
5.0	.109	.150	.182	.206	.223	.237	.249	.258	.266	.271
6.0	.077	.109	.135	.155	.170	.183	.194	.202	.210	.215
7.0	.055	.079	.101	.119	.132	.143	.153	.161	.170	.174
8.0	.040	.059	.076	.091	.104	.113	.121	.128	.135	.140
9.0	.029	.044	.058	.070	.081	.088	.095	.102	.108	.113

Cobalt-60

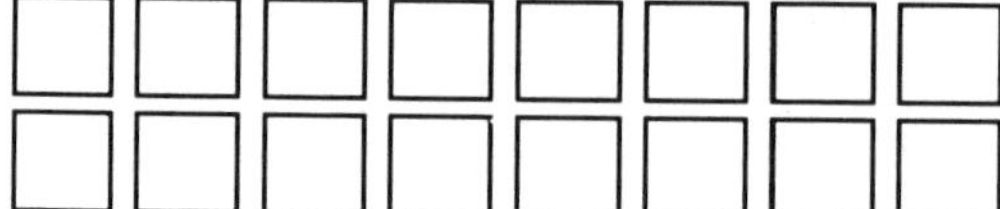 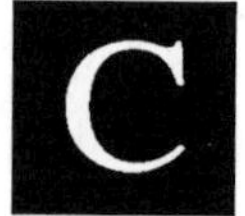

Calibration Sheet
Cobalt - 60
Picker C-9
UAB Dept. of Radiation Oncology
Buildup Depth = 5 mm
Timer correction: Subtract .011 minutes from calculated time
Date pertains to cGy/min. at d_{max} in maxiphantom
-To find cGy/min. for specified field, multiply field size factor by 10 x 10 cm field size dose rate-

DATE	10 x 10 cm DOSE RATE
3/81	138.0 cGy/min
4/81	136.5
5/81	135.0
6/81	133.5
7/81	132.1
8/81	130.6
9/81	129.2
10/81	127.8
11/81	126.4
12/81	125.0
1/82	123.6
2/82	122.3
3/82	120.9

Cobalt-60 (UAB)
Depth Dose Fractions

d = depth (cm)

Field Size (cm)

d	4	6	8	10	12	16	20	24	28	32	36
0.5	1.000	1.000	1.000	1.000	1.000	1.000	1.000	1.000	1.000	1.000	1.00.
1	.974	.974	.976	.984	.986	.983	.984	.985	.985	.985	986
2	.913	.926	.927	.936	.939	.943	.944	.945	.946	.946	.949
3	.854	.871	.876	.889	.891	.900	.900	.903	.905	.906	.909
4	.797	.818	.827	.841	.844	.854	.855	.859	.862	.864	.867
5	.740	.765	.778	.794	.797	.807	.810	.815	.819	.821	.824
6	.686	.714	.730	.748	.749	.761	.766	.771	.776	.779	.783
7	.635	.664	.682	.701	.704	.716	.723	.730	.734	.737	.742
8	.587	.617	.637	.655	.660	.673	.682	.689	.694	.698	.704
9	.543	.572	.593	.613	.617	.632	.642	.651	.656	.660	.667
10	.501	.529	.552	.572	.577	.593	.605	.614	.619	.624	.631
11	.462	.490	.513	.533	.540	.556	.569	.578	.584	.589	.596
12	.487	.453	.476	.497	.505	.521	.535	.544	.550	.556	.562
13	.384	.419	.442	.462	.471	.488	.503	.512	.518	.524	.530
14	.364	.388	.410	.430	.439	.457	.472	.481	.487	.493	.499
15	.336	.359	.381	.400	.410	.427	.443	.453	.459	.465	.470
16	.311	.332	.354	.373	.382	.400	.416	.425	.431	.437	.442
17	.287	.303	.328	.347	.357	.374	.390	.400	.406	.412	.417
18	.266	.285	.305	.323	.332	.350	.365	.375	.382	.387	.392
19	.246	.264	.283	.301	.310	.327	.342	.352	.359	.365	.370
20	.227	.244	.262	.280	.288	.305	.320	.330	.337	.343	.348
21	.209	.226	.243	.260	.268	.285	.299	.309	.316	.323	.327
22	.192	.209	.225	.242	.249	.265	.279	.290	.297	.304	.308
23	.177	.193	.209	.224	.232	.248	.260	.272	.279	.285	.290
24	.163	.179	.193	.208	.215	.231	.243	.254	.261	.268	.273
25	.151	.166	.180	.193	.200	.215	.227	.238	.245	.252	.256
26	.140	.154	.166	.179	.186	.200	.213	.223	.230	.236	.240
27	.130	.143	.154	.166	.173	.186	.199	.209	.216	.222	.226
28	.121	.133	.143	.155	.161	.174	.187	.196	.203	.208	.212
29	.113	.124	.133	.143	.150	.163	.175	.184	.190	.195	.200
30	.105	.115	.124	.133	.140	.153	.164	.172	.178	.183	.188

Field Size (cm)

4	6	8	10	12	16	20	24	28	32	36

Monitor Factor

4	6	8	10	12	16	20	24	28	32	36
.958	.976	.990	1.006	1.024	1.059	1.087	1.105	1.117	1.126	1.130

Cobalt-60 (UAB)
Tissue Maximum Ratios (TMR)

d = depth (cm)   Equivalent Square

d	4	5	6	7	8	9	10	11	12	13	14
.5											
1	1.000	1.000	1.000	1.000	1.000	1.000	1.000	1.000	1.000	1.000	1.000
2	.985	.986	.991	.988	.988	.992	.996	.998	.998	.997	.996
3	.946	.952	.960	.958	.960	.966	.970	.973	.974	.974	.976
4	.905	.915	.925	.926	.929	.936	.942	.946	.946	.947	.950
5	.862	.876	.888	.891	.896	.904	.911	.917	.917	.918	.922
	.819	.835	.849	.854	.861	.871	.879	.885	.885	.887	.890
6											
7	.775	.793	.809	.816	.825	.836	.845	.852	.852	.853	.856
8	.732	.751	.769	.777	.787	.799	.808	.816	.817	.819	.821
9	.690	.710	.728	.738	.749	.762	.772	.780	.782	.784	.786
10	.650	.671	.689	.699	.711	.725	.736	.746	.748	.750	.752
	.612	.632	.650	.661	.673	.688	.701	.711	.714	.716	.719
11											
12	.575	.595	.613	.625	.637	.652	.665	.677	.680	.684	.687
13	.542	.560	.578	.590	.602	.617	.631	.643	.648	.652	.656
14	.510	.527	.544	.556	.569	.583	.598	.610	.616	.621	.625
15	.479	.496	.513	.525	.537	.551	.565	.578	.585	.591	.594
	.451	.467	.483	.495	.507	.521	.535	.547	.555	.561	.565
16											
17	.424	.440	.455	.467	.479	.493	.506	.518	.527	.533	.538
18	.399	.415	.430	.440	.452	.465	.479	.491	.499	.506	.511
19	.375	.391	.405	.415	.426	.439	.452	.464	.473	.480	.485
20	.352	.368	.382	.391	.402	.414	.426	.438	.448	.455	.460
	.331	.345	.358	.367	.378	.390	.402	.413	.423	.431	.435
21											
22	.310	.323	.336	.346	.357	.368	.379	.390	.400	.408	.412
23	.291	.303	.316	.326	.336	.347	.357	.367	.377	.385	.390
24	.273	.284	.296	.306	.316	.327	.336	.346	.356	.364	.368
25	.256	.265	.277	.288	.298	.308	.317	.326	.336	.344	.348
	.240	.249	.261	.271	.281	.290	.299	.307	.317	.324	.328
26											
27	.226	.235	.246	.256	.265	.274	.282	.290	.299	.306	.310
28	.213	.222	.233	.241	.250	.258	.265	.273	.282	.289	.293
29	.201	.210	.220	.228	.236	.244	.250	.257	.266	.273	.276
30	.190	.199	.208	.215	.222	.230	.236	.242	.250	.257	.261
	.180	.188	.196	.203	.210	.217	.223	.229	.236	.242	.246

Field Size (cm)

4	5	6	7	8	9	10	11	12	13	14

Monitor Factor

4	5	6	7	8	9	10	11	12	13	14
.952	.961	.970	.977	.984	.992	1.000	1.009	1.018	1.027	1.035

d	15	16	17	18	19	20	21	22	23	24	25
.5	1.000	1.000	1.000	1.000	1.000	1.000	1.000	1.000	1.000	1.000	1.000
1	.995	.995	.996	.996	.996	.996	.996	.996	.996	.996	.997
2	.976	.978	.978	.979	.979	.979	.978	.978	.979	.979	.979
3	.952	.954	.956	.957	.956	.956	.955	.956	.956	.957	.958
4	.924	.927	.929	.930	.930	.930	.929	.930	.930	.931	.932
5	.892	.896	.898	.901	.901	.901	.901	.902	.902	.903	.905
6	.859	.862	.866	.869	.870	.871	.871	.872	.873	.874	.876
7	.824	.828	.832	.836	.838	.839	.840	.842	.844	.845	.846
8	.789	.794	.798	.803	.805	.807	.810	.812	.814	.815	.817
9	.755	.760	.765	.770	.773	.776	.779	.782	.784	.786	.788
10	.722	.727	.733	.738	.742	.745	.749	.752	.754	.756	.758
11	.691	.696	.701	.706	.710	.714	.718	.722	.724	.726	.728
12	.660	.665	.670	.675	.679	.684	.688	.692	.695	.697	.700
13	.629	.634	.640	.645	.650	.655	.659	.664	.666	.669	.671
14	.599	.604	.610	.615	.620	.625	.630	.625	.638	.640	.643
15	.570	.575	.581	.586	.591	.597	.602	.607	.610	.613	.615
16	.542	.548	.553	.558	.564	.570	.575	.580	.583	.586	.589
17	.516	.522	.527	.532	.538	.543	.549	.554	.557	.560	.563
18	.490	.495	.501	.506	.512	.517	.523	.528	.532	.535	.537
19	.465	.470	.475	.480	.486	.492	.498	.503	.507	.510	.513
20	.440	.446	.451	.456	.462	.467	.473	.478	.482	.485	.488
21	.417	.422	.427	.432	.438	.444	.449	.454	.458	.461	.464
22	.394	.399	.404	.409	.415	.421	.426	.431	.435	.438	.441
23	.373	.378	.383	.387	.393	.399	.404	.409	.413	.416	.419
24	.352	.357	.362	.367	.372	.377	.383	.387	.391	.394	.398
25	.333	.338	.342	.347	.352	.357	.362	.367	.370	.374	.377
26	.314	.319	.324	.329	.333	.338	.343	.347	.351	.355	.358
27	.297	.302	.307	.311	.316	.320	.324	.329	.333	.337	.341
28	.281	.286	.290	.295	.299	.304	.308	.312	.316	.320	.324
29	.265	.270	.275	.280	.284	.288	.292	.297	.301	.305	.309
30	.251	.256	.261	.266	.270	.274	.278	.282	.286	.290	.294

Field Size (cm)

	15	16	17	18	19	20	21	22	23	24	25

Monitor Factor

	15	16	17	18	19	20	21	22	23	24	25
	1.044	1.053	1.061	1.068	1.074	1.080	1.085	1.090	1.094	1.098	1.100

d	26	27	28	29	30	31	32	33	34	35	36
.5	1.000	1.000	1.000	1.000	1.000	1.000	1.000	1.000	1.000	1.000	1.000
1	.996	.997	.997	.997	.997	.997	.997	.998	.998	.998	.998
2	.979	.980	.980	.981	.981	.981	.981	.982	.982	.982	.983
3	.958	.959	.960	.961	.961	.962	.962	.962	.963	.963	.964
4	.933	.934	.935	.937	.937	.938	.939	.939	.940	.940	.941
5	.906	.907	.908	.910	.911	.912	.913	.913	.914	.915	.916
6	.877	.878	.880	.882	.883	.884	.885	.886	.887	.888	.889
7	.848	.849	.851	.853	.854	.855	.856	.857	.858	.860	.861
8	.818	.820	.822	.824	.825	.827	.828	.829	.830	.831	.833
9	.789	.791	.793	.795	.796	.798	.799	.800	.801	.803	.805
10	.760	.762	.764	.766	.769	.770	.771	.772	.774	.775	.777
11	.730	.733	.735	.737	.739	.741	.742	.774	.746	.748	.750
12	.702	.704	.706	.709	.711	.713	.715	.716	.718	.720	.722
13	.673	.676	.678	.681	.683	.686	.687	.689	.690	.692	.694
14	.645	.648	.650	.653	.656	.658	.659	.661	.663	.665	.677
15	.618	.621	.623	.626	.629	.631	.633	.634	.636	.638	.640
16	.591	.594	.597	.600	.603	.605	.607	.608	.610	.612	.614
17	.566	.569	.572	.575	.578	.580	.582	.584	.586	.588	.589
18	.540	.543	.546	.549	.552	.555	.557	.559	.561	.563	.565
19	.515	.519	.522	.525	.528	.531	.533	.535	.537	.539	.541
20	.491	.494	.497	.501	.504	.507	.509	.511	.513	.516	.518
21	.467	.470	.474	.477	.480	.483	.486	.488	.491	.493	.496
22	.444	.447	.451	.454	.458	.461	.464	.466	.469	.472	.474
23	.422	.425	.429	.433	.436	.439	.442	.445	.448	.450	.453
24	.401	.405	.408	.412	.415	.419	.421	.424	.427	.429	.432
25	.381	.385	.388	.392	.396	.399	.401	.404	.406	.409	.411
26	.362	.366	.369	.373	.377	.380	.382	.385	.387	.390	.392
27	.344	.348	.352	.355	.358	.362	.364	.366	.369	.372	.374
28	.328	.331	.335	.338	.341	.344	.347	.349	.352	.354	.357
29	.312	.316	.319	.322	.325	.328	.330	.333	.335	.338	.340
30	.297	.301	.303	.306	.309	.312	.314	.317	.319	.322	.324

Field Size (cm)

	26	27	28	29	30	31	32	33	34	35	36

Monitor Factor

	26	27	28	29	30	31	32	33	34	35	36
	1.103	1.107	1.110	1.113	1.115	1.117	1.119	1.120	1.121	1.122	1.123

Clinac-4

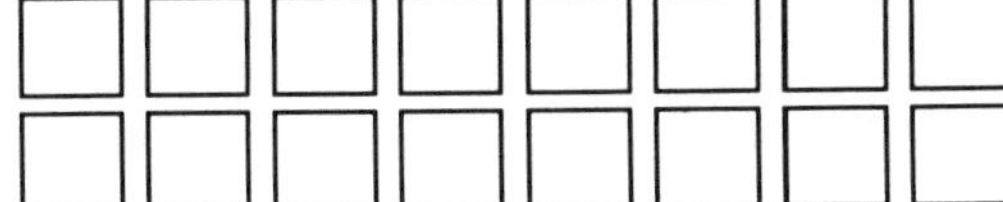

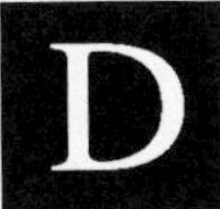

Depth Dose Fractions
Clinac-4 - 4 MV photon

d = depth (cm)   Field Size (cm)

d	3	4	6	8	10	12	14	18	22	26	30
0	.135	.147	.172	.199	.224	.249	.273	.323	.371	.409	.430
1	1.000	1.000	1.000	1.000	1.000	1.000	1.000	1.000	1.000	1.000	1.000
2	.943	.947	.952	.955	.956	.958	.960	.962	.962	.963	.963
3	.884	.891	.900	.905	.908	.912	.915	.919	.922	.924	.925
4	.825	.834	.847	.855	.861	.867	.872	.876	.880	.882	.885
5	.766	.776	.795	.807	.814	.822	.827	.833	.839	.842	.844
6	.713	.723	.745	.759	.769	.778	.784	.792	.799	.803	.805
7	.660	.673	.698	.713	.724	.735	.741	.751	.759	.764	.767
8	.613	.627	.653	.670	.682	.694	.701	.712	.721	.727	.730
9	.570	.584	.607	.627	.641	.654	.662	.674	.684	.690	.694
10	.530	.544	.568	.587	.601	.615	.624	.639	.648	.655	.657
11	.492	.506	.530	.549	.564	.576	.588	.605	.614	.622	.627
12	.456	.470	.494	.514	.529	.543	.554	.572	.583	.591	.596
13	.421	.436	.461	.480	.496	.511	.522	.540	.551	.560	.565
14	.390	.404	.429	.449	.465	.480	.491	.509	.521	.528	.535
15	.362	.375	.400	.419	.435	.450	.462	.479	.491	.500	.506
16	.335	.348	.372	.391	.407	.422	.434	.452	.464	.473	.478
17	.310	.323	.347	.366	.381	.395	.408	.425	.438	.447	.451
18	.289	.301	.323	.342	.357	.371	.382	.401	.413	.421	.426
19	.269	.280	.302	.320	.335	.348	.359	.378	.389	.397	.403
20	.251	.261	.281	.299	.314	.327	.338	.356	.368	.377	.382
21	.232	.243	.262	.279	.293	.307	.317	.334	.348	.357	.362
22	.215	.226	.245	.261	.275	.288	.297	.314	.328	.335	.340
23	.199	.210	.227	.244	.258	.270	.279	.295	.308	.316	.321
24	.184	.195	.213	.228	.242	.253	.262	.278	.290	.299	.304
25	.173	.182	.200	.214	.226	.237	.247	.262	.274	.282	.287
26	.161	.171	.186	.200	.212	.223	.232	.247	.259	.267	.271
27	.151	.159	.174	.189	.199	.210	.218	.233	.244	.250	.255
28	.140	.149	.163	.176	.187	.198	.205	.220	.230	.237	.241
29	.131	.138	.152	.164	.175	.185	.192	.207	.217	.223	.228
30	.122	.129	.142	.154	.165	.173	.181	.194	.204	.211	.215

Field Size (cm)

3	4	6	8	10	12	14	18	22	26	30
				Equivalent Square						
.927	.941	.965	.984	1.00	1.010	1.020	1.036	1.047	1.054	1.059

Tissue Maximum Ratio
Clinac-4 - 4 MV photon

d = depth (cm)   Field Size (cm)

d	4	6	8	10	12	14	18	22	26	30
1	1.000	1.000	1.000	1.000	1.000	1.00	1.00	1.00	1.00	1.00
2	.970	.975	.978	.978	.981	.983	.985	.986	.987	.987
3	.934	.943	.949	.952	.956	.959	.964	.967	.970	.971
4	.894	.908	.917	.923	.930	.935	.940	.945	.948	.951
5	.851	.870	.884	.892	.901	.907	.914	.921	.926	.928
6	.811	.833	.849	.861	.872	.879	.889	.898	.903	.908
7	.770	.797	.815	.828	.841	.849	.861	.871	.879	.883
8	.733	.760	.781	.796	.810	.820	.834	.846	.853	.860
9	.697	.724	.746	.762	.779	.790	.806	.820	.828	.834
10	.662	.689	.712	.729	.746	.759	.778	.793	.802	.809
11	.629	.655	.678	.697	.714	.727	.750	.767	.776	.786
12	.595	.622	.647	.666	.685	.699	.722	.741	.753	.762
13	.562	.591	.616	.636	.655	.671	.694	.714	.727	.737
14	.531	.560	.585	.607	.626	.643	.667	.687	.701	.710
15	.503	.531	.557	.577	.597	.614	.640	.657	.674	.685
16	.475	.503	.528	.549	.570	.586	.614	.634	.649	.668
17	.448	.477	.502	.524	.543	.559	.587	.608	.625	.637
18	.426	.452	.477	.498	.518	.534	.561	.584	.606	.611
19	.404	.429	.454	.475	.495	.510	.537	.561	.577	.588
20	.384	.407	.430	.452	.472	.487	.515	.538	.554	.568
21	.362	.386	.408	.429	.448	.465	.491	.513	.532	.547
22	.342	.366	.389	.408	.427	.443	.468	.491	.510	.524
23	.322	.347	.369	.388	.407	.423	.448	.469	.488	.501
24	.303	.328	.350	.368	.387	.403	.427	.449	.468	.482
25	.290	.312	.334	.351	.368	.383	.409	.430	.450	.462
26	.274	.297	.316	.333	.350	.365	.391	.412	.432	.445
27	.260	.281	.300	.319	.335	.349	.373	.394	.414	.426
28	.247	.268	.286	.302	.319	.333	.357	.378	.386	.409
29	.235	.252	.271	.286	.302	.317	.339	.360	.378	.392
30	.222	.240	.257	.272	.289	.303	.324	.344	.361	.374

Field Size (cm)

	4	6	8	10	12	14	18	22	26	30
Equivalent Square	.941	.965	.984	1.00	1.01	1.02	1.036	1.047	1.054	1.059

206

Clinac-18

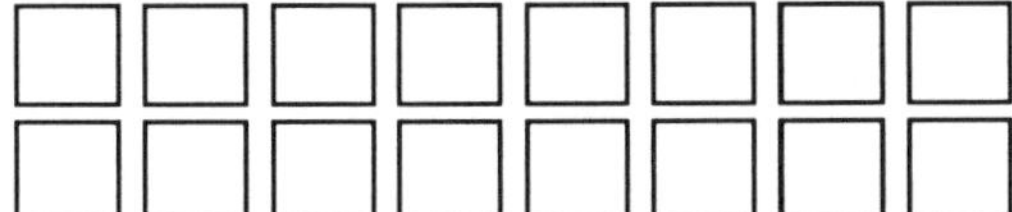
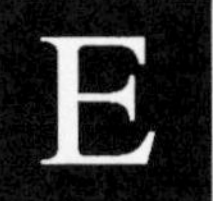

Clinac-18
10 MV photon
Tissue Phantom Ratios normalized at 2.5cm

d = depth (cm) Field Size (cm)

d	4 x 4	6 x 6	8 x 8	10 x 10	14 x 14	18 x 18	22 x 22	26 x 26	30 x 30	35 x 35
0	.061	.037	.110	.130	.169	.211	.250	.285	.316	.351
1	.868	.877	.886	.895	.915	.936	.947	.956	.958	.958
2	.992	.996	.996	.996	.997	.999	1.003	1.003	1.002	1002
2.5	1.000	1.000	1.000	1.000	1.000	1.000	1.000	1.000	1.000	1.000
3	.994	.995	.996	.996	.994	.993	.995	.995	.986	.986
4	.969	.972	.975	.977	.975	.975	.977	.977	.978	.978
5	.939	.948	.951	.952	.954	.956	.958	.960	.960	.962
6	.909	.916	.925	.926	.930	.933	.939	.939	.941	.943
7	.878	.890	.899	.902	.909	.912	.919	.921	.922	.923
8	.847	.862	.874	.877	.887	.892	.897	.901	.903	.903
9	.819	.834	.848	.852	.865	.870	.880	.882	.884	.884
10	.790	.810	.821	.828	.842	.850	.854	.861	.865	.867
11	.758	.773	.798	.804	.816	.827	.834	.841	.845	.847
12	.722	.746	.764	.781	.790	.804	.815	.822	.825	.828
13	.700	.721	.738	.755	.768	.781	.793	.801	.806	.809
14	.674	.697	.713	.731	.746	.758	.773	.733	0.788	.791
15	.651	.673	.690	.707	.724	.738	.752	.762	.767	.768
16	.629	.649	.667	.684	.702	.718	.732	.742	.747	.749
17	.606	.627	.645	.662	.681	.697	.711	.723	.728	.731
18	.584	.606	.624	.641	.660	.676	.691	.704	.709	.712
19	.563	.685	.603	.620	.639	.657	.672	.681	.691	.694
20	.542	.564	.582	.600	.618	.638	.654	.664	.673	.678
21	.523	.543	.561	.580	.599	.619	.636	.646	.655	.659
22	.504	.523	.540	.561	.579	.601	.619	.629	.638	.642
23	.486	.505	.521	.541	.560	.582	.600	.611	.621	.625
24	.468	.488	.503	.523	.542	.563	.582	.593	.604	.608
25	.452	.471	.487	.505	.525	.545	.568	.576	.587	.591
26	.436	.454	.470	.489	.528	.525	.548	.560	.571	.575
27	.427	.438	.454	.473	.492	.512	.531	.544	.554	.559
28	.404	.428	.437	.458	.477	.497	.515	.528	.538	.542
29	.390	.408	.423	.441	.460	.480	.498	.511	.520	.524
30	.377	.394	.410	.425	.444	.464	.481	.494	.503	.507

Monitor Factor (mf)

mf	.922	.958	.981	1.000	1.026	1.048	1.061	1.072	1.077	1.078

* Skin doses measured without shadow tray
**Fields greater than 35 x35 cm measured at 2 meter SAD

Glossary

Atomic Number (of an element) - the number of electrons in the atom or, equivalently, the number of protons in atomic nuclei.

Betatron - an electron accelerator which produces x-rays and electrons. The electrons are accelerated in a circular path due to a changing magnetic field.

Bolus - tissue-equivalent material which is placed on the skin at the involved site to even out the irregular surface of a patient in order to present a flat surface normal to the incident beam. This gives rise to acceptable uniformity of dose within the target volume.

Bremsstrahlung - the fundamental process occurring when a fast moving electron experiences a force as a consequence of its near collision with the positively charged nucleus of an atom; as a result the electron is diverted from its straight line path.

Buildup bolus - a bolus layer which is equal to the buildup thickness to bring the absolute maximum dose onto the skin surface. This thickness depends upon the energy of the photon beam.

Buildup depth - the depth for a single field at which the maximum absorbed dose occurs.

Cesium-137 - a radioactive nuclei with a half-life of 30 years and a dominant gamma-radiation energy of 0.66 MeV.

Collimator - in a linear accelerator, it consists of two pairs of continuously movable upper and lower jaws. It provides a rectangular opening ranging from 0 x 0 cm to the maximum field size of 40 x 40 cm or less at a distance 100 cm or 80 cm from the source. The collimator is made of either lead or tungsten blocks.

Compton Effect - a phenomenon in which a photon interacts with an electron to produce a scattered photon with lower energy and a scattered electron.

Coulomb (C) - unit of electric charge.

Density (of a substance) - its mass divided by its volume.

Dose - the energy deposited per unit mass.

Dose buildup - the maximum absorbed dose for a single field which occurs at a specific depth depending on the beam energy.

Dose profiles - profiles of dose distribution versus distance from the central ray at fixed depths.

DSD - diaphragm to skin distance.

Electron - the lightest elementary particle with a mass of 9.11×10^{-31} kg and charge of -e, where $e = 1.60 \times 10^{-19}$ Coulomb.

Electron equilibrium - when as much electrical charge due to ionization migrates into the region as out of it.

Electron Volt (eV) - the energy acquired by an electron accelerated through a potential difference of one volt.

Equivalent square - it is possible to define an equivalent square of a rectangular field on a non-square field which produces the same percentage backscatter as the equivalent square field under consideration.

Ergs - unit of energy equal to 10^{-7} joule.

Exposure - a measure of the ability of radiation to ionize air. It is useful for x and gamma ray photons with energies up to about 3 MeV.

F-factor - the cGy to roentgen conversion factor.

Flattening filter - a device constructed usually of lead, tungsten, steel, uranium, aluminum, or a combination of these. It is inserted in the beam; its function is to yield a dose distribution essentially constant from the center of the radiation field to the edge.

Gamma Rays - energetic photons emitted by radioactive nuclei of the atom.

Gray - one Gray is equal to one joule of energy absorbed per kilogram of mass; also equal to 100 rads.

Half-value layer (HVL) - the thickness of a material which reduces the incident intensity of the beam to half its initial value.

Horns - are created by introducing the flattening filter in the beam. This is due to overcompensating near the surface in order to achieve flat isodose distributions at greater depths.

Integral dose - the total energy absorbed from the beam by an irradiated medium.

Intensity - energy per unit area per unit time.

Ion chamber - an instrument for measuring the ionization produced as a result of interaction of radiations with medium.

Joule (J) - the unit of energy and work in the metric system; equal to 1 kg-m^2/s^2.

Kilogram (Kg) - the unit of mass in metric system. One kilogram weighs 2.21 lbs.

kVp - the peak excitation voltage. The prefix k has a numerical value of 1000.

Lens - a transparent object that can produce an image of an object placed in front of it.

Maxiphantom - an extended phantom large enough so that if it were larger it would make no difference in the dose measurement at the point of interest. Sometimes referred to as a "semi-infinite" phantom.

Miniphantom - a sphere of tissue equivalent medium surrounding a point of interest (or around the air volume of a measuring chamber) of just sufficient size to provide buildup at the center.

MV - a unit used to express the energy of a photon beam; equal to one million volts.

Neutron - a particle which is electrically neutral and with mass of 1.675×10^{-27} kg.

Pair Production - results from annihilation of a photon to an electron-positron pair. Pair production occurs only in the presence of another nucleus. The threshold energy for pair production is 1.02 MeV, which is twice the rest energy of an electron or a positron which is equal to 0.511 MeV.

Penumbra trimmers - extensions which may be placed on the collimator jaws which move with the jaws, and when in place define the field edge.

Penumbra - a region characterized by a rapid decrease in dose as one moves outward from the center, where only a portion of the source is contributing primary radiation.

Photoelectric Effect - occurs when a photon interacts with an atom which results in emission of an electron. The emitted electron is also called a photoelectron. In the photoelectric effect the incident photon is completely absorbed.

Photon - a particle with zero mass which travels with speed of light (3.0×10^8 m/sec).

Pi Mesons or Pions - discovered in 1935 by the Japanese physicist, Yukawa. He proposed that the strong nuclear interaction could be explained as a result of certain particles exchanged between nucleons. These particles are called pions. The name pion is a contraction of the name Pi-Meson. Pions are charged or neutral. Those with a positive charge (+e) or negative charge (-e) have rest masses of 273 times the electron mass. The neutral pions have rest masses of 264 times the mass of an electron.

Positron - the antiparticle of the electron with positive charge +e.

Protron - a particle that carries a positive charge of +e and mass of 1.673×10^{-27} kg which is 1836 times that of the electron.
Rad - absorbed energy of 100 ergs of energy per gram (or 0.01 J/ kg) of medium.

Roentgen (R) - unit for quantitatively measuring the amount of exposure. It is equal to 2.58×10^{-4} coulombs of charge liberated per kilogram of air under electronic equilibrium.

Scattering foil - a thin metal foil (made of copper, lead, tantalum, tantalum plus brass, etc.) inserted into a high energy electron beam. It reduces the energy of electrons passing through it and gives rise to some secondary radiation to cover larger area.

SDD - source to diaphragm distance

"Semi-infinite" depth (in a phantom) - when enough water depth exists behind the measured points so that if more depth were added it would not affect the measurements.

"Semi-infinite" medium (in a phantom) - implies a considerable amount of tissue-like medium beyond the last point of interest.

Shutter or Timer Correction - the time that the source is in motion at the beginning or end of the treatment. This time should be used to correct exposure rate or dose rate.

Skin-sparing - with photon beams at megavoltage energies the surface dose is small and buildup occurs at a maximum depth beneath the surface; this results in a skin sparing effect. The skin sparing effect of megavoltage radiation is one of the main advantages of using higher energy beams in radiation therapy.

Source-skin distance (SSD) - source to surface distance.

Teletherapy - external beam treatments in which the source of radiation is a distance away from the patient.

Umbra - a region characterized by a gradual change in dose, always decreasing. It has a much smaller value than in the center or penumbra. It receives no primary radiation except that transmitted through the collimator, usually less than one percent.

X-Rays - photons (electromagnetic waves) emitted when fast electrons impinge on matter (i.e., tungsten, copper, etc).

Index